The International Library of Psychology

MAN AND HIS FELLOWMEN

Founded by C. K. Ogden

The International Library of Psychology

SOCIAL PSYCHOLOGY
In 7 Volumes

I	Personal Aggressiveness and War	*Durbin et al*
II	The Psychology of Politics	*Eysenck*
III	Dynamic Social Research	*Hader et al*
IV	The Group Approach to Leadership-Testing	*Harris*
V	Co-operation, Tolerance, and Prejudice	*Lowy*
VI	Man and His Fellowmen	*Lowy*
VII	The Symbolic Process and its Integration in Children	*Markey*

MAN AND HIS FELLOWMEN

Modern Chapters on Social Psychology

SAMUEL LOWY

Routledge
Taylor & Francis Group
LONDON AND NEW YORK

First published in 1944 by
Routledge
2 Park Square, Milton Park, Abingdon, Oxfordshire OX14 4RN
711 Third Avenue, New York, NY 10017

First issued in paperback 2014

Routledge is an imprint of the Taylor and Francis Group, an informa business

British Library Cataloguing in Publication Data
A CIP catalogue record for this book
is available from the British Library

Man and His Fellowmen
ISBN 0415-21121-2
Social Psychology: 7 Volumes
ISBN 0415-21134-4
The International Library of Psychology: 204 Volumes
ISBN 0415-19132-7

ISBN 13: 978-1-138-87577-7 (pbk)
ISBN 13: 978-0-415-21121-5 (hbk)

CONTENTS

PREFACE

The abundance of psychological knowledge, with its interconnected fields and the fruits they have borne, has not yet sufficiently enriched social life. The blame for this belongs solely to the scientist. It is he who is called upon to place his findings and conclusions before the public, and to draw the attention of statesmen and administrators to theories and facts of potential importance to social advance. It must be admitted that he has done this inadequately.

It is impossible to expect the thinking but busy politician to study the complicated and conflicting theses of the different psychological schools and authors, and to extract from them what is proven and what is of the first importance in planning a better social future. Any constructive activity of value requires that its promoter should possess a theoretical foundation appropriate to his particular interests and activities. Just as the life of the individual, to be satisfactory, requires a firm ideological background, so the social worker should possess a systematized knowledge of the established theories and scientific results which should constitute a constant basis from which to start in the approach to a variety of problems.

In this small volume the author wishes to describe certain aspects of individual and social life in terms of psychology. He does not aim at the full and detailed presentation of every problem dealt with by various experts in social psychology; this, though 'scientific', would doom his endeavour to failure. He wants to be understood by every educated reader, and to influence the hearts and minds of social workers and all who are concerned for social reconstruction.

In training—to employ an illustrative analogy—a joiner, we should do well to teach him as much as possible about the physical qualities of wood, and about certain chemical processes that enable industry to adapt wood to its purposes. But we should not waste time by teaching him all the intricacies of the chemistry of the cellulose of which wood consists, or all the processes through which wood is being utilized as a component material in other branches of industry, outside his future trade. The same principle holds good for the psychological presentation of problems connected with social planning. Selective treatment is obviously not only necessary for our practical purpose, but the only 'scientific' one for the end in view.

This work does not aim at outlining concrete proposals for future social reforms. Yet it is concerned only with the concrete issues of social life, and with those only in so far as State organizations can contribute to progressive improvement in the social sphere. This book is thus meant to be read, and read, perhaps, more than once, by the general reader interested in social reform ; and especially by the active worker in that field. It aims at giving an up-to-date and, as far as possible, an unbiased presentation of social facts as revealed by the psychologist's analysis.

Emphatically this book disclaims finality. It should prove suggestive to some readers, and others will certainly be provoked to criticism of its inevitable shortcomings and of controversial statements. It is the author's sincere desire that others, far more gifted and learned and experienced than he happens to be, should continue the work on similar lines, to further the great cause of human progress in so far as the psychological approach to human problems can directly affect the world of realities.

There is especially one shortcoming that might be charged against the author. The reader will not find in this work the usual mass of quotations from other authors, or the many references customary in scientific publications. The general background of the discussion is admittedly that of contemporary analytical psychology. But the particular suggestions made in this book proceed in the main from first-hand knowledge gained and conclusions arrived at, in the course of fifteen years of continuous thinking on social psychology during the analytical treatment of individual patients. The present volume is based mainly on lectures delivered by the author in the years 1930-36 in Bratislava (the capital of Slovakia), at the request of various societies interested in science and social progress; and especially on two lectures delivered in recent years at the Czechoslovakian Centre in Manchester. All the problems dealt with in this volume are presented in the light of the latest views advanced by modern writers on social psychology.

Though this volume is not based on quotations and references, the author is fairly confident that his views are not peculiar to himself; he is sure that he does not stand alone in his interpretations or in the suggestions he ventures to offer. It is inevitable, of course, that he should express some views which may dismay many well-intentioned people of traditional outlook. He wishes only to state that he sincerely regrets this necessity.

The author advises the reader to turn first to the few pages comprising the Closing Remarks. It is hoped that this will facilitate the reader's approach to the work and his ready grasp of the case for some of the views advanced. The author's chief aim has been to point out the significance of the 'social process'[1] in all the fields of human existence dealt with in his present work; and he wishes to direct the reader's attention primarily to this particular aspect of his exposition of the various spheres of individual, family, and communal life.

[1] See page 56.

ADDENDUM TO AUTHOR'S PREFACE

THE Introduction is written by Mr. Herbert Read, formerly Professor of Fine Art in the University of Edinburgh, whose recent book, *Education through Art*, is an admirable attempt at utilizing modern psychological conceptions for the analysis, on broad lines, of the artistic or creative faculty in its relationship to the social aspect of the individual. He thus represents that trend of our times which endeavours to put into practical service, for the benefit of the masses, the results of scientific research.

I am grateful to Mr. David Redwood, tutor of Political Science at the Extramural Department, University, Manchester, who read the manuscript and made a few valuable suggestions. I am indebted to Mr. E. W. Dickes for his substantial help in preparing the MS. for the press. I am also much obliged to the W.E.A., Urmston branch, Manchester, for inviting me to lecture on Social Psychology. In the course of my work with the students I had opportunity to substantiate some of my results arrived at through observation and psycho-analyses in Czechoslovakia, in a social environment in many respects different from that of Great Britain.

The few personal case-histories and psycho-analyses cited in this book took place in various countries on the Continent, and with one exception (Ch. XVII) more than a decade ago. The participators therefore cannot be identified. S. L.

February 1944.

INTRODUCTION

When Dr. Lowy surprised me by asking me to write an introduction to this book, my first reaction was to beg him to seek someone who carried more weight in the scientific world, to which he himself belongs. As a layman who has dabbled in psychology, I am a little suspect in learned circles, and my advocacy might do more harm than good to a doctor's reputation. But Dr. Lowy argued very convincingly that he had written his book primarily for the lay public, and that I, as a layman who had shown some hunger for the fruits of psychology, was in a position to point out to what extent this book is satisfying.

Psychology is the science which has the most direct impact on our daily lives. Other sciences affect our meal-times or our working hours, our power over nature or our understanding of the physical universe. But psychology is with us all the time, for it is the science of our minds, of our feeling, thinking and dreaming minds. It is, if any science can be, the clue to our happiness, and in this respect the psychologist has to a great extent taken over the functions of the priest. But in spite of this fact, psychology remains for the ordinary man a learned mystery expressed in an incomprehensible jargon. For that reason, if for no other, it has had so far singularly little effect on the general behaviour of mankind.

There have been attempts in the past to summarize or popularize the various schools of modern psychology, and some modern psychologists have become popular figures, lecturing to large audiences all over the world and receiving the devotion of innumerable disciples. Any man with a cure for sick souls can, of course, set up as a prophet : and there are so many sick souls about today that he is sure to find a large following. But such success is always won at the cost of a simplification which distorts the truth. The human mind is an intricate system of compensations and balances, of actions and reactions, all of which have to be taken into the total view. To seize on some detached scrap of information about this system and use it as a clue to our own or (more probably) our friends' behaviour is neither helpful nor ingenious. It is merely exasperating. How often, for example, we are told that some individual is suffering from 'an inferiority complex', and how rarely does our informant understand, not only what the psychologists understand by that term, but how inadequate it is to describe the likely mental disposition of a particular individual. Modern psychology is thoroughly *dynamic* in its conceptions of personality, but the popular use made of it is confined to a few fixed labels.

Many difficulties beset the path of anyone who, like Dr. Lowy, would attempt to present the public with a synoptic view of modern psychology which is not merely comprehensive but also practical. He cannot carry the simplification of the terminology too far: words like repression, inhibition, sublimation, fixation, identification, etc., are precise and definable terms whose meaning must be learned just as we expect to learn the meaning of terms like atom, electron and molecule in physics. But psychology is not an exact science to the same degree that physics is. Different physicists have different hypotheses, but there is a general agreement on the use of a scientific method, and the terminology of this method is universal. Two physicists might have different theories of molecular structure, but they would use the same terms to explain their theories to each other. But if two psychologists set out to explain their theories of the structure of the mental personality they might make use of completely different systems of terminology. Sometimes the terms mean the same thing, and sometimes the same terms are used for different things: and so rapid has been the development of psychology during the last fifty years that some terms change their meaning, even within the same psychological school.

Dr. Lowy does not claim, so far as I am aware, any supreme degree of impartiality. He is himself a pupil of Stekel, but in his important work of *The Psychological and Biological Foundations of Dream-Interpretation* he advanced far beyond his master's achievements in that particular field. Dr. Lowy has made a deep study of all the leading psychologists of our time, not least of Freud: and he is a practising analyst of wide experience both on the Continent and here in England. I cannot myself discover that he has any particular bias, except towards the scientific truth: and certainly in this volume he has striven to give, not a personal view, but the general body of facts which emerges from a correlation of the leading schools of modern psychology.

These facts are of immense importance for every individual. They affect his personal happiness, his marriage, his relations to his parents and his children, his work and play, his activities as a citizen and his metaphysical cravings. There is much that the ordinary man and woman can learn from this book which would immediately affect their conduct and ensure a greater degree of happiness. Dr. Lowy pursues these implications into the family circle, the school, the church and right into the political structure of society. Much that he has to say—much that modern psychology has to say—has a direct bearing on the immediate problems of war and peace. He finds, justly enough, that in the application of psychological theses to the interpretation of social facts, " science has so far failed to produce many workers of an *eclectic* type ", with the result that " insufficient attention is paid by men of concrete activity in politics and administration to psychological aspects and suggestions ". How true this is was obvious in the so-called realistic outlook which most politicians adopted before the war towards the growth of fascism. They treated as an economic or at best as a political problem, to be solved by compromise and appeasement, what was essentially a problem of social psychology, amenable only to psychological treatment. But then, as Dr. Lowy admits, we do not yet possess " a sufficient number of individual psycho-therapists who are of the type that is fitted to work on the lines of *social prevention* ". I would myself suggest that we do not yet possess a technique of social analysis (*phylo-analysis*, as Dr. Trigant Burrow has called it) which would enable us to pass beyond the methods and scope of individual analysis. No number of psycho-analysts, working all the time on an indefinite number of individuals, would prevent the development of group conflicts and mass neuroses. It is the group itself that must be treated.

It is in this connexion that I find myself in somewhat sharp disagreement with Dr. Lowy. He says (page 128) that " men will remain essentially what they have always been : humanly weak, but capable of intellectual and moral achievements, *if* guided and compelled. But this latter will always remain the task of an external superior factor, of an organized legal *State-authority*, in combination with a suitable '*public opinion*'." And in several other contexts he invokes the aid of this external ' State-authority '. But what is this ' State ', and from whence does it derive its extraordinary authority ? In concrete terms, is it ever anything but the dominance of specific economic interests : and otherwise is it ever anything but an abstraction which creates a fundamental disunity between social and organic processes ? The whole tendency of social psychology should be to create an inner accord between individual morality and spontaneous group activities. That it can be done has been demonstrated, not only in various primitive societies, but in contemporary experiments such as that conducted by Dr. Scott Williamson and his assistants at the Peckham Health Centre. The way lies through reciprocity and mutual aid, not through coercion and external authority. The authoritarian state is only to be understood as a projection of the neurotic symptoms of the individual: as an objective embodiment of the power to which, under the compulsion of unconscious masochistic drives, the individal seeks to submit himself. It is a myth, appropriate perhaps to a certain stage of human development, but a stage which, we may hope, is undergoing its dying convulsions in the present world conflict. Elsewhere Dr. Lowy shows himself so deeply aware of the importance of creative and spontaneous activities, even in their collective aspect, that I fail to see why he should in this one particular pay his tribute to a compulsive abstraction. I would rather suppose that he speaks his real mind in these words :

> " Deep down in everybody's psyche there is a simple, uncomplicated, unsophisticated soul, easily satisfied by the necessary amount and necessary kind of nourishment, sunshine and air, peace and ease, and by a fairly friendly, sympathetic, and loving environment."

That, at any rate, is the ' elementary personality-layer ' which lies well within the scope of the social psychologist, and if his technique can be effective at this layer, there will obviously be no need for those complicated superstructures which man has evolved out of his poverty, envy and separateness.

HERBERT READ.

CHAPTER I

THE NEED FOR SOCIAL PSYCHOLOGY

1. HOMO SAPIENS likes to conceive of himself as a being fully capable of looking after himself. He likes also to believe that he automatically acquires full knowledge of all that he needs to know in relation to his own nature and to his earthly needs and obligations. Thus it is generally assumed that the individual will be safe in behaving according to his own natural, untutored judgment, and in simply employing his common sense and discretion in the decision of what to do and how to do it, and what not to do and why not to do it.

Men have achieved so much in the course of human history, have displayed such proof of intellect, skill, and power, that it is difficult to challenge this claim that man knows by nature all that he need know of the essentials of living. There have, indeed, been many manifestations of reluctance to acknowledge the necessity of the psychological analysis of man, of his mind, and of his deeper motives of action. There is a very intelligible reason for this. Man is expected to behave in his daily life as his thought prompts him to do; but this seems to presuppose that the conscious sector of his mind is his whole mind. To appreciate that the mind is in fact a very complicated instrument, so much so that a large sector of it needs special examination for its functioning to be observed at all; to realize that the conscious motivation of feeling and action is not the sole and whole source of man's behaviour—this is bound to be more or less unpleasant. It may well produce a state of mind comparable to the embarrassment felt when one is faced for the first time in one's life with an anatomical atlas showing on different plates the various parts of the body: one plate shows all the muscles, another the blood-vessels; a third shows the open abdomen with its contents, and so on.

In the presentation of man's life and his actions in novels or historical works, it is supposed to be the whole and full man who acts, who strives and performs heroic and admirable deeds, who fights in attack or defence, rules or revolts, builds or destroys, creates and invents, and enjoys the beauties of nature and art. But the case is not so simple as this. The deficiencies of our social organization are too obvious, the need for a more skilful and better planned advance is too manifest, and the necessary 'finishing touches' in our social structure seem beyond possibility of accomplishment merely by employing the knowledge and the conceptions of human nature which were deemed sufficient in the past.

Just as the moulding and utilizing of our physical environment, resulting in all the refinements of the technical aids to living, in the modern ways of utilizing wood and steel and dyes and drugs and electricity, has been greatly extended and intensified by exact research, so further social progress may well be made possible by more minute study of man's nature.

It is true that a great deal of fruitful work has been done in many spheres by past generations ; many accomplished personalities did emerge from the mass, many really decent citizens and parents moved about the stage of life, carrying on their callings and enjoying their days, though not in possession of the advantages of our modern minute investigation of individual and social psychology. Thus it is easy to understand the inclination of so many leading figures in scientific and public life to look askance at the advocacy of increased attention to the psycho-sociological aspect and to the possible psychological background even of minute features of life. Many people tend to say : "Look at me and my like : are we so very lacking in moral fibre and human efficiency ? And we are, as you know, products of the old ways of looking at things, and believe in fighting our way through the difficulties of life with the aid simply of our natural endowments."

It has never been possible, however, to interfere with the continuous progress of social organization ; and all the scientist wants to do, and has to do, is to continue to search for new facts and causal relationships, in the hope that the additional knowledge thus gained may prove of ultimate if not of immediate service to it. It has so often occurred in the past that considerations and suggestions put forward have failed at first to be appreciated, but later have been independently arrived at and resubmitted and then hailed as of the utmost practical value. The ideas of human equality before the law and of the right to freedom of religious conviction were not always accepted as self-evident as they are today. The ideas of communal feeding[1] and of the socialization of the medical services are similarly not propounded for the first time in our own day. To take another field of research : the existence of electrical waves moving through infinite space had been postulated several years before concrete experience of them was gained through the invention of wireless

[1] Cf. Popper-Lynkeus, *Phantasien eines Realisten.*

communication. And how many thinkers dreamed, through all the ages, of human flying, until at last it has become a concrete reality! All these things, long no more than aspirations, were destined to ultimate achievement.

In view of such past experiences as these, any research aiming at social improvement, and any presentation of its results or implications for the information of thinking people, deserves a hearing ; even if its immediate usefulness is not apparent to the uninitiated.

2. There is no agreement on the question of what is in need of review and reform in our society. Many problems raised by authors and discussed in stormy meetings appear to a substantial proportion of the public to be merely topics for enthusiasts. It is noteworthy that a great number of middle-class persons in secure positions, especially persons holding administrative or executive posts in the Civil Service and those belonging to the organizing class in industry and business, feel satisfied with the existing social organization. It is not so much their financial situation as their social position and their justified sense of their social significance that account for their satisfaction ; but the sense of economic security also counts. Under the influence of their personal situation these 'efficient' members of society are too ready to assume that what applies to them should be applicable to millions of others. They like to assume that general conditions are more or less satisfactory, only needing periodical overhaul. Their subjective outlook prevents them from fully realizing how few enjoy the privileged positions they occupy, and how many millions are without their opportunity of satisfying their personal ambitions. And many a psychologist who today is keenly interested in social problems will admit that in the past his own interest was confined to the cure of individual cases. The tragic events of the last decade have made many of us more fully alive to the importance of a more extensive and more courageous social planning.

It appears to the social psychologist that far more individuals could be given a freer and securer existence, and better opportunities for the appreciation of all that is human and beautiful, than ever before in human history, if we only had the courage to break away from many traditional conceptions.

Increased spontaneity in the life of the individual is certainly the aim of all enlightened and progressive social endeavour.

And though it may sound paradoxical, men can be forced into such spontaneity. We shall have frequent occasion to refer to the *social process*, to those environmental influences which mould men's character and behaviour. So many trends which appear today to be part of human nature and impossible to eliminate, so much restlessness and aggressiveness and pursuit of false values, are simply the unsatisfactory mental functioning produced by historical environmental defects, or manifestations of unhealthy nerves. And planned and even forcible measures, by suppressing some inclinations, may easily pave the way to increased mental harmony. Such results are frequently secured in individual psycho-therapy. The patient learns to give up infantile, and consequently deeply ingrained, emotional tendencies ; and he may gain in exchange more harmony, added efficiency in carrying out his work, and increased enjoyment of the gifts of nature.

3. There are two ways of planning the future and making, as it were, prophetic statements and suggestions. The realist proper views the immediate future, and proposes concrete steps which proceed clearly from the conditions of the immediate past. In the main these follow directly from institutions already in existence, improving them by means of additional or corrective measures. Such proposals quickly find more or less general acceptance as obviously sound and useful.

But there is another way of thinking about the desirable future. It is comparable to the scientific method of the physicist, who through his knowledge of the ' mathematical formula ' of development may foresee further stages of progress. To the uninitiated, or to the ' realist ', this method, when applied to social research, may seem Utopian and in no way warranted by existing conditions. Yet this is the method not only of the physicist but of the physician. He too, if well experienced in diagnosis, is, as a rule, equally good at prognosis ; he may visualize the future course of a pathological process, and its probable final outcome, by drawing conclusions from his knowledge of the nature of the illness and from the specific constitution of his patient.

A similar way of looking into a more distant *social* future is no less realistic. And suggestions on these lines may well have some influence even on current concrete proposals. A courageous society, and its leaders, whilst carrying out reforms of immediate urgency, may allow, within the framework of its plan, for improvements possible only at a later time.

The author has in mind above all, in this connexion, such an extension of public education and enlightenment on the absolute essentials of life, and on its intricate complexities, as the present generation has not yet the courage to permit; though nearly everybody, in his secret heart, admits that various private and social deficiencies are due to a lack of such advanced education. Yet, within any new framework for future educational reform, new plans could already be envisaged, to enable the next generation to introduce compulsory education on such problems, for instance, as the social sense and its disorders, the psychology of marriage and of its difficulties, the emotional and physical aspects of sexuality, and so on.

4. Every generation is, in one respect, in a more favourable position than its immediate predecessor or, indeed, any earlier generation: it knows the outcome of some of the unfulfilled hopes of the past. No previous generation, however enlightened, could have foreseen the things that are possible today. And the hopes of the past of preventing the horrors of war, and of allaying the misery that has been man's lot in all ages, simply by continuing to rely on the accepted social methods of the past, may safely be dismissed as illusory. We now know for certain, we know better than any past generation could do, that the progress of human civilization must not be left simply to free individual initiative and to ethical propaganda appealing simply to the individual.

We have not been poor, indeed, in the highest ethical principles. We are used in Europe to regarding the Judaeo-Christian Bible as the sole source of all ethics, though it is well known that other civilizations also produced systems of humanitarian and self-restrictive ethics. But let us consider our own Bible and its teachings. The idea that all men originate from a *not yet racial* (not Jewish but universal) Adam prepares the way for the conception of the equality of men. The biblical ethics require that we shall love our fellowman as we love ourselves [1]; that we shall not wreak vengeance nor bear any grudge [2]; that we shall love the foreigner and do him no wrong.[3] The biblical principles denounce selfishness,[4] theft,[5] exploitation of the weaker

[1] Lev. xix. 18. [2] Lev. xix. 18. [3] Lev. xix. 34; Deut. xxiv. 14, 17.
[4] Lev. xix. 10; Deut. xxiv. 20-21. [5] Lev. xix. 11.

and oppression of the employee[1]; they denounce unrighteousness in judgment,[2] whether through respect for the wealth of the rich or undiscriminating consideration for the poverty of the poor ; they condemn slander and slander-propaganda,[3] condemn passive murder through holding aloof from a fellow-being in mortal danger[4]; and repeat several times the warning to consider especially the mentality of the foreigner, because of his relative social isolation and weakness.[5] And the injunctions of Jesus add the love of the enemy (hardly possible in practice, though a sublime theoretical principle) ; advocate to repay wrong by good,[6] and similar principles of extreme humility—and command His idealistic ‘ communism ’.[7]

Really, if the continuous and untiring efforts of the clergy to instil these biblical principles have so failed to eradicate brutality and aggression, and to replace them by humanity, justice, respect for the equality of men, and lovingkindness, what can we expect from a continued reliance simply on the ethical appeal to the spirit and conscience of man?

We must not be unjust. Most of the progress in the conception of social justice, and in its materialization, during the many centuries of human history is linked closely with the spiritual influence of religion on men's minds. The penetrating intensity of the hopes and fears of a metaphysical kind, instilled by religious dogma, have greatly developed the sense of ethical obligations in man's attitude toward his fellowmen ; and even in modern times this ethical insight into good and evil operates substantially enough. Indeed, no organized and legally maintained social order could attain any high standard if it were not met half-way by men's own genuine concern for social justice. It is rather in its insufficient practical result that this concern has proved its inefficacy. It has been too much a matter of every man's free will. It is bound to continue to fail of effect in the future in the absence of new kinds of measures.

[1] Lev. xix. 13 ; Deut. xxiv. 14. [2] Lev. xix. 15. [3] Lev. xix. 16.
[4] Lev. xix. 16. [5] Exod. xxiii. 9 ; Deut. xxiv. 17, 22.
[6] Matt. v. 44, and Matt. v. 39, 40, 46. Cf. Exod. xxiii. 4, 5.
[7] Acts ii. 44 ; iv. 32, 34, 35.

CHAPTER II

AFTER THE SECOND WORLD WAR

1. One day the war will have come to an end. The strain of continuous danger from the air and of painful restrictions and burdensome conditions, weighing now so heavily on the soldier, and to a lesser degree, but still substantially, on the civilian, will have gone. And with this relief many things will go, and others will emerge. Many phenomena of the weary years of war, due to the simple fact of severe strain, will change or disappear. Tendencies of a more individualistic character, likes and dislikes, aspirations and resentments, kept under for so long by the overriding effect of the war on man, will inevitably emerge again.

Men have always been dissatisfied because of the little they have, and the much more they have not ; and with a good measure of objective justification. And from ancient times men have sought a simple, an over-simple, explanation for what is not quite right in the small world of their existence. They generally found that they had not what they ought to have because one or more of their neighbours enjoyed the little or much more that fate and fortune had given them.

The human mind has so many things to do that it tends, just as the body does, to devote as little effort as possible to each of them. Simplest explanations may be demonstrably wrong, unjust on the face of it, no contribution at all to the solution of concrete difficulties ; yet the simplest of explanations is preferred to any objective search for true reasons and remedies.

The easiest way has always been to grudge the friend's good fortune, to envy the neighbour's success and to think : "Why, he is just as insignificant as I am" ; or, "I am just as good as he is ; it is unfair that I should not have what he has." There has always been much envy of the great and powerful, too, but as a rule it has never been so deep or so keenly felt as the grudge against the little man next door.

To him has been attributed the blame for all that is wrong. And if he happened to be so unfortunate as to be different in any way, of a different denomination or race or nationality, then his neighbours were pretty sure that the very air he breathed, the water he drank, and the bread he ate, ought to have belonged to them, and unfairly reduced their own share.

2. In recent decades there has been much discussion of social reform. This implies the admission that the ‘ root of the evil ’ is not the individual’s better success : the task to be tackled is universal, a ‘ social ’ one. But the simple mind, and even the educated man’s mind, works on a more primitive level under the influence of ill-success and want. The simple mind prefers the ‘ concrete formula ’ that enables it to envy and to hate a particular group of people, in accordance with primitive tendencies which are repressed only by culture.

The deeper psychological reason for this preference is probably, at least in part, the fact that if the envied fellowman could be attacked without much risk, and robbed of what he has, even uprooted from his home and his land, his supplanter’s problems would find a comparatively easy solution. There seems to live in the unconscious recollection of man the certain knowledge that in primitive times, and not infrequently in the so-called Middle Ages, that simple solution was within reach. If our present nightmare does not deceive our senses, that simple solution seems within reach even in our own day, and far more real than some of the scientifically-worked-out theories of modern social progress, the materialization of which is so costly, so difficult, so hypothetical. In short, to the simple man, with his aggressive weapon at hand, or at least ready in his subconsciousness, the sight and thought of his defenceless fellow-creature suggests a more concrete step toward mending the deficiencies of his material condition than any idealistic conception which has in view the whole of society.

And this outlook will inevitably re-emerge in the minds of the masses, all over the world, after the present involuntary equality, enforced only by the war, has lost its sole source, the external pressure of the law amid our present necessities. True, there will be more talk of social reform, of universal justice, and of communal principles than in any previous period of human history. There will even be more genuine goodwill in the hearts of tens of thousands. But the more elementary social forces will once more breed envy and hatred of the heterogeneous. And this narrow outlook will tend again to set limits to the right to life and dignity of the stranger who dwells within the gates. A narrow outlook is essentially indicative of an arrested development of the emotional spheres, and is expressive of an only limited functional freedom of the mind. Hence the inclination of the narrow-minded person to limit the field of human tolerance and collaboration to a small number of fellowmen ; he is unable spontaneously to embrace a wide circle of society with his faculty of love and appreciation.

CHAPTER III

THE IMPOSSIBLE HAS BECOME POSSIBLE

THERE will be freedom once more—more freedom of private and public speech than at present. And the hatreds, the various 'anti-propagandas', will flourish again. I am afraid that hatred propaganda may flourish with far greater intensity than twenty to thirty years ago. For it is impossible to make non-existent the influence on men's minds of the extraordinary and appalling events of the present war and the decade preceding it. The automatic functioning of the mind in judging and conceiving is always substantially influenced by the particular quality of past experiences, which leave their traces in the deeper layers of the psyche. All the brutality of the Fascist ideology on the one hand, and on the other the horrifying necessities of the present warfare, have shifted the barriers that existed in men's minds in the past between the possible and the impossible.

Things never dreamed of as possible in the past are now daily occurrences. The life of every civilian, of every child, is exposed to daily risks, and millions of people are dealt with as cattle, with no respect for life or limb ; and all this has become 'possible', imaginable, even for the kindest and justest and most humane. But things which have once become conceivable may constitute thereafter a continuous temptation to the 'repressed beast' in the minds of the most cultured of men.

It may prove far more difficult than in the past to overcome elementary aggressive, envious, selfish tendencies. The actual possibility of dethroning established law, of disregarding the bonds of solemn promises and agreements, the possibility of easily and entirely getting rid of fellow-beings, cannot be eradicated from the consciousness of our generation. Many a man will feel that he is acting rather heroically, not merely doing his elementary duty, in holding aloof from the unscrupulous gangs of the future.

Unless this radically altered mentality of mankind is met by planned counter-measures, legal and educational, human society may be caught by new surprises. The moral standard in feeling and behaviour of the individual and of the masses is based on constant 'automatized' sentiment. It is not the immediate situation and the momentary intellectual response to it that determine the quality of moral behaviour. It is the quality of the subconscious moral standard that decides inciting or deterring. Poor, very poor, is the moral dependability of an individual for whom nothing, or not much, is really horrifying and unthinkable, and for whom the most atrocious things may only be inexpedient. The world does not yet realize what happened to us in the last decade, what happened to us owing to the inertia of those who for a time were not directly concerned by the bestiality from which a less fortunate but large section of humanity were suffering.

That the formerly impossible has become not only possible but a natural way of behaving in a considerable part of man's world—this is a loss, a cultural regression, a menace which will long take toll of mankind's happiness and of his progressive dynamism.

CHAPTER IV

HATRED AND AGGRESSION

1. Much has recently been written on the psychology of hatred. It was, in fact, the much praised, and even more criticized, Sigmund Freud who stated that aggression is not simply a defensive reaction and a means of guaranteeing life and vital needs : man is by nature aggressive, cruel, destructive, independently of all necessary and useful aims.[1]

It is usual in the abstract sciences, of which psychology is one, to start with definitions of the concepts to be discussed ; and there is, indeed, plenty of room for enlarging on the theoretical psychology of hatred, aggression, and destructiveness. But the author wishes to confine himself in this volume to the realm of practical life, and will only indicate certain theoretical details which may bear some relevance to concrete problems of social life.

Hatred may be described as intra-psychic[2] *aggression.* It is a mental attitude, highly charged with emotion, toward an object, a principle, or a living being ; and the indulgence of this feeling

[1] Freud, *Civilization and Discontent,* 1929.

[2] That is to say, aggression carried out only *within* the mind, but experienced as strongly as if occurring in actuality.

seems to satisfy the desire for actual aggression and to serve as a substitute for it. In the world of his fantasies the hating person is able to multiply his attacks on the hated object, and even to destroy it again and again ; and from this point of view the satisfaction-value of hatred is more extensive than that of a factual single attack. The conception of hatred and love as related sentiments is not merely a sophisticated psycho-analytical conception. We know from life, without the help of scientific psychology, that the most burning hatred, and even hatred resulting in serious attacks, may be developed and felt against persons originally loved or appreciated. This may happen if the beloved or admired person meets his fellowman's craving for reciprocation with rejection or simply with cold indifference.

To hate anyone in the fullest sense always implies a measure of emotional interest in him. And this very fact seems, we think, to prove a particular explanatory theory about hatred founded on prejudice. This explanation states that the prejudiced person essentially hates something *in his own subconsciousness* ; but he projects this ' evil within him ' on to another person, and vents his hatred on that external person. The original object of such hatred is, therefore, one's own personality, or part of it ; and consequently the hating interest, though overtly and consciously directed toward the innocent hated fellowman, *derives from the naturally substantial interest in one's own personality.*

2. There is, apparently, a natural inclination in everybody, though varying in degree, to hate. It seems that hatred is the emotional response to anything unsatisfactory, if the unsatisfactory condition can be connected with a person or thing that can be held responsible for it. The human mind tends to connect the subjective unsatisfactory condition with a person or thing outside itself—a person or thing that could be regarded as to blame for it, however remotely. And since there are in the course of life plenty of reasons for feeling dissatisfied, the opportunities of developing hatred are frequent. In a later chapter I shall explain how a great number of individuals, owing to an innate constitutional insufficiency within their own psycho-nervous system, frequently feel ill at ease, and dissatisfied with things or with themselves ; and accordingly their psyche readily produces hatred resulting in a craving for attacks ; though they do not admit or even realize the disharmony within them.

The sense of dissatisfaction produces other things besides

hatred. Every striving, every activity, the urge, for instance, to make a better living and to get on better in the world, are the result of the sense of lacking something, the result of some degree of dissatisfaction. Hatred arising from dissatisfaction is probably indicative also of something else, of a sense of helplessness in the face of undesirable facts or conditions. But there must also be a natural tendency toward overt aggressiveness, sufficient to make the individual react with hatred in response to his intra-psychic dissatisfaction.[1] In the case of such psycho-nervous difficulty in coping with processes deep within the mind, the element of helplessness is clearly inevitable, since nobody can escape from his own self. Certain neurotic symptoms, such as fits resembling epilepsy and compulsory actions in obsessional neurosis, are supposed to be the outcome of internalized hatred. These symptoms are fed by hatred which was aroused by people in one's environment, but which has been directed back toward the self.

The disproportionate hatred aroused in many individuals by small slights or petty conflicts is clear evidence of a general inclination toward hating. And the perennial sentiment of malicious joy (German : '*Schadenfreude*') at the misfortune of a person whose only fault was to inflict some small and even unintentional injury on one, is also indicative of an intrinsic need for hatred in man. The noble sport of hunting—not killing for food—clearly reveals the general aggressive and destructive tendencies in man. And the glorification of war and singling out of adversaries to be attacked and defeated, of enemies who, until the attack was made, were not adversaries at all—this well-known attitude of past centuries, centuries so glorified in books of national history, is sheer aggressiveness and lust for destruction.

3. But I should like to draw the reader's attention to more peaceful and more justified activities of civilized man. When the great or distinguished individual has to fight for his principles in science, in art, or in politics, and an overt victory has been won, then look at him, and at his followers ; or look into your own heart if *you* happen to be just such a great and distinguished leader ; and ask yourself : " How much of this gratification is due to the victory of the truth, and how much of it is merely satisfaction at

[1] 'Intra-psychic' denotes here that the primary causation of the dissatisfaction originates within the mind.

the defeat of the others, mingled with malicious joy at their discomfiture in defeat and at the suffering this brings them ? "

And too often in the past we have seen teachers teasing, and even punishing, small children for some minor neglect of their 'duties', or for displaying natural, human, but 'indecent' tendencies ; torturing them by words, and even physically, to such an extent that the calm onlooker can only conclude that " This man is not merely administering corrective justice, he is not simply concerned for the future well-being of his pupils; he enjoys being a bit cruel and tyrannical with the weak and helpless ".

It has always been said that Government offices, local and central, are for the citizens ; that they are instituted to make decisions for the citizens, for the sake of just organization and fair distribution of rights and duties. When, however, the individual citizen, that 'atom' of the organized State, thinks he ought to receive a certain permit or licence as a means for improving his personal condition, for bringing, perhaps, a little beauty into his toilsome, humdrum life, he may find at times that his 'case' is dealt with by an official whose natural inclination is to refuse. The official may be in the habit of subjectively interpreting the regulations, their wording, their reference to dead paragraphs, so meticulously, so boggling at minutiae, that he is sure to find some legal ground for rejecting the application. Not infrequently a subordinate official of this type is even considered by his superior as 'very efficient'. What else is at work in the minds of such trustees of human rights, of human lives and happiness, than the unconscious primitive desire for aggression against those who are subject to their guiding and deciding power ?

It might be useful if millions of citizens in various countries could be given at least an occasional opportunity to witness and investigate such cases of bureaucratic arbitrariness. They would find that in many of them no harm would have been done to the State or the community, and no great burden imposed on the Exchequer, by acceding to the request, which might have meant so much to the applicant if granted; and the refusal of which may not only have subjected him to unnecessary restrictions, but may in some cases have seriously interfered with the basic aims of his life, frustrating the only conditions of his individual happiness and success.

It could do no harm—though it would hardly be practicable —if the same millions of common citizens could have an opportunity to look *analytically* into the mind of such an official, into the deeper subconscious motives for his decisions, into that abyss of destructive individualism which is present in everybody, but which in theory is the very opposite of the principle that is expected to be the intellectual and emotional background of the activities of a Civil Servant. If once discovered and sufficiently realized, a great deal of such unconscious or unadmitted destructiveness might be effectively countered by the increased alertness and criticism of the general public.

We must not exaggerate the quantitative significance of this special field of possible subconscious aggressiveness. I am sure, indeed, that the cases in which humane, sympathetic motives, also of a subconscious and emotional character, guide the decisions of a Civil Servant are at least as numerous as those in which aggressive complexes are at work. The essential point for our present discussion is that the Civil Servant makes his decisions on behalf of the State and community, acting in the name of that impartial justice and care which the community wishes to see given to its individual members by its organs.

4. The same not entirely conscious aggressiveness may influence all human activities where one individual has to deal with any sphere of the life of another. The manager in a factory, the sergeant in the army, the nurse in a hospital, the warder in a prison, even the doctor treating suffering and helpless patients or the teacher of tender children or the distinguished scientist examining students, all could do with some general psychoanalytical knowledge related to this problem ; and also with some knowledge about the depths of their own mind. They should all learn to acquire the caution exercised by the surgeon in approaching and carrying out his highly important but risky task.

This problem of aggressiveness, whether resorted to for the achievement of concrete aims and gains, or simply for the sake of subjective satisfaction, this problem of 'innate badness', is as old as human history. The fight against it is as ancient as is the realization by man that there is an absolute need for universally valid ethical principles. And to this day no detail of this problem, no suggestion to meet it, can be so small or so trite as to justify its disregard. Anything that is brought forward with the aim of facilitating social research, of discovering new avenues for social improvement, deserves a hearing and earnest consideration.

This ancient problem of unmotived, autochthonous human aggressiveness merits special attention at the present time, amid the tendencies to more and more comprehensive control and planning and organization of human life. The planners and controllers, the executors of this new, more or less communized life, cannot be other than average human beings, with the natural inclinations of such beings. They are chosen individuals of those masses who feel and think and act under the motivation of their own psyche. The more extensive the future field of the State control that aims at safeguarding a more even distribution of rights, means, and burdens, and at removing the opportunities for excessive individual exploitation, the more we have to face the risks involved in this extension of official rights. Almost everything that affects human life and happiness may in future be controlled and officially regulated. The consequent emergence of purely individual, subjective forces of bias, dislike, and sheer aggression in the course of official activities, may become a more serious problem than in past times, when there still remained to the private individual so many opportunities of remedying the deficiencies of life by his independent initiative. Certainly the scientific study of aggressiveness, and of human motivation in general, deserves and demands more study than ever before in human history.

CHAPTER V

INTERFERENCE WITH OTHERS' LIVES

1. MOST of the satisfaction and pleasure attained in the life of average people is made possible only through their fellow-beings. And, similarly, the greatest amount of suffering—mental, but physical too—comes from the actions and omissions of fellow-beings. In a social system where the scope of individual enterprise is almost unbounded, there is a possibility for a limited few to gain enormous wealth, and with this they have access to many means of improving their condition and protecting themselves from various troubles. Naturally no amount of wealth will make up for a lack of family happiness, or for the lack of the desired type of private cultural environment. But the mass of average people depend, in almost every sphere of their lives, on others—

on the degree and the manner in which these others fulfil their elementary human duties toward them.

A concrete instance may ease the reader's approach to this problem. But first a few preliminary remarks. There is, as we know, such a thing as syphilitic infection. And there is, on the other hand, in young men such a thing as sexual desire. It is true that when a man succeeds in his fight against his desire until he is able to marry his partner for life he is usually not exposed to the risk of infection. But the avoidance of pre-marital intercourse is not so simple, not so universal, and even not so desirable in every case, as it seems to be in the wishful thinking of the well-meaning moralist.

First, a few words about this last aspect of undesirability. It is perfectly true that people not infrequently marry at an age and under economic conditions which should have made marriage unthinkable ; they do so nevertheless, essentially because they wish to legalize the satisfaction of their urgent erotic desires. For this step they have to pay—and their children still more—with years of misery, with a life of disharmony or financial difficulties, or usually both. Much to be commended are purity of life and chastity of mind, and fortunate is the lot of those who are able to start and maintain their sexual life within a relationship of mutual appreciation, love, and the social security of legality. Yet we know very well how the socially enforced chastity of a great number of people is anything but the experience of a lofty, spiritualized frame of mind ; actually it consists in the sense of a futile fight, with consequent depression and irritability, and in living in a world of their fantasies, which is by no means a world of beauty and mental cleanliness. In this state of inward tension so many love-affairs start that lead later to marriage without genuine love, marriage necessitated merely by social conventions ; and so many extraconjugal pregnancies occur, compelling hasty marriage—and the consequences in both groups are only rarely enviable. Frequently, owing to the lack of mutual love and respect, the temptation to a change may become very strong. All this implies even more harm to the children of such unions.

There always have been, and always will be, young men who know little about the results of social statistics and of research into sexual psychology, and who decide on their own account to satisfy their sexual needs when the tension is high and the opportunity cheap and easy. And with this fact goes, in our society, the possibility of venereal diseases. Be it noted at this point that a person may have had illegitimate pre-marital intercourse only once, and yet may contract syphilis through it; and if not completely cured he will be virtually an outcast for his lifetime. And another person may be so fortunate as to lead a life of unbridled lust for many years, especially when acquainted with the means of preventing V.D., and may end up as a decent married man, unsuspected and free from all blame. Only when, owing to some minor neurosis, he is compelled to undergo an analysis, may his past be established without a shadow of doubt.

And now for the concrete instance. A man who unfortunately had contracted syphilis in his youth had married later, and married happily. At the outbreak of war he had to go into the army. Owing to the great stress of war conditions his latent syphilis of the brain became acute; he was discharged from the army and soon after died in hospital. The widow, a woman of an outlook and understanding above the average, wanted to know how far life in the army had hastened the outbreak of the disease of the brain, and how far she could therefore claim compensation. The first thing to do in such cases is to get the authorities to order a post-mortem examination by a trained pathologist and to ask his opinion on his findings from the condition of the organs. In this case the medical officer whose duty it would be to inform the authorities happened to be a woman of high moral principles, very helpful in general life, but in this particular case irritable and unsympathetic. Finally, under persuasion, and probably owing to gaining a better insight, she did what she was required to do. But before she fought through to this decision, and while still acting under revulsion and putting official difficulties in the way of social justice, she burst out: "I cannot understand these people; first they contract syphilis and then they make such a fuss about themselves." As a short conversation following this revealed, the contemptuous remark sprang from moral condemnation of all extra-conjugal intercourse. Now, the poor widow knew quite well about her husband's past contraction of syphilis, and had fully condoned it. What she did deplore was that he had not been treated soon enough or thoroughly enough. This implied a certain accusation against the social conditions that had resulted in this case, and no doubt in many others, in insufficient concern for the effectual treatment of venereal diseases. Finally, it will not have escaped the reader that it was in fact the poor patient who had been so 'shameless' in the past as to contract his disastrous disease; whilst the 'fuss' was made after his death by his even poorer wife, who only wanted the help from the State to which she was entitled.

2. It is evident how substantially prejudice or revulsion in a person in authority may interfere with the elementary rights of man. There is, in fact, hardly any field of administration in which semi-conscious or fully conscious motives of prejudice and aggression may not enter into and vitiate the process of judgment, decision, and action.

It might well be inferred that all persons in authority should undergo periodical tests of their general human fitness and their professional capacity to carry on their occupation, and as to the possession of a certain minimal objectivity in making decisions affecting the lives of others. Unfortunately it is difficult even to imagine how such a plan could be satisfactorily carried out.

3. Dr. Stekel, the Viennese psycho-analyst, who published so many deeply interesting books on the social and educational aspects of the experience gained during his psycho-analyses, told of a judge who was well known for his merciless severity in punishing indecent assaults on children. He habitually imposed the maximum sentence, even if cruelly disproportionate. One day he committed suicide because, as was suspected with good reason after his death, the temptation was so strong in him to commit the very offence he had been so zealous throughout his career in trying to stamp out.

The present writer was personally acquainted with a clergyman who was very strict and even malevolent toward his younger colleagues who would put on lay clothes and attend lively social gatherings. He denounced them for their irreligious modernism and did them a good deal of harm. Yet those well acquainted with his own past history well remember how ardently he used to court girls whilst a student at a very strict theological college; and even earlier, how unbridled and undisciplined a youngster he had been. His friends, anxious to explain away his intolerance, used to talk of his nerves. He made many journeys, frequently for unknown ends—to all appearance simply for the sake of distraction. I know from analyses carried out by myself, as well as from cases recorded in published works, that people of strict morals, who with difficulty repress their polygamous tendencies, like travelling, for the reason, admitted or not, that it stimulates their imagination of possible adventures, and this travelling and day-dreaming may satisfy their mind. I do not know whether this was so in the clergyman's case. Restlessness and the impulse to travel may certainly have other backgrounds. But I think we should keep this possibility in mind in this man's case, in view of his past record as a youngster and a student, so different from his strait-laced attitude in later years.

Dr. Stekel taught us also that many parents are very strict about the friendships of their children with members of the other sex, from a sort of envy and jealousy. They want to have their children's whole affection,[1] and are even jealous because the time of their own youth and potential adventures has gone. I beg the reader to believe at least that such possibilities do exist. Occasionally—not very often—I hear similar admissions from my patients ; only, it is true, when I have guessed that this was their attitude from the study of their dreams, and when they are being hard pressed to search themselves and to speak frankly. The persistent fight of adults against the habit of masturbation in the young is only partly due to traditional ignorance and misconceptions of the true nature of this phenomenon. Their horror derives a substantial degree of its intensity from a similar unconscious begrudging [2] on their part. We psycho-analysts are fairly sure about the existence of this factor in sexual education ; though we are aware of the difficulty of attaining the understanding of the wider public for this statement. At the same time the moral factor in this anti-sexual fight must not be denied or overlooked. Parents wish to see the absence in their children of a biological urge which is the source of so many difficulties in the world of adults.

I know also of a comparatively young father who is very religious because he himself was very strictly brought up, but who at the same time frequently plays with atheistic and revolutionary ideas, and even expresses them openly in the presence of his children. He is very strict with his children, and especially with his only daughter. She, however, tends to free-thinking ; besides, she has fallen in love with a quite decent youth of her age (16) who, like her, is a free-thinker. One day her father went for a walk with her in a park and tried to persuade her to stay at home, to be religious, and especially to give up her 'boy'.

[1] Janet stated something similar. He observed a great number of cases of parents warmly attached to their children up to the age of fifteen, but later hating them so much as to force them to leave home—in jealousy of the children's awakening independent emotional interests.

[2] German : *Sexualneid.*

The scene ended—in the open park—with the father mercilessly beating his tender young daughter, from anger, and—I am able to say, for I know him—from jealousy. It should be added that a year before this incident the father had been involved in an intrigue. He and his wife were compelled for some months to leave their home, and while they were away, though his wife was living in the same town with him, staying with her relatives (he could not afford to rent a house), he was making overtures to a young girl and trying to persuade her to enter into intimacy with him. In the end he was found out; the girl herself denounced him "to make it hot for him".

4. The following incident occurred in a small town where the present writer used to live in his youth. He had the opportunity at a later period to psycho-analyse two people closely concerned with the story. There was a certain government office, the head of which was a quiet, urbane man, thoroughly efficient in the discharge of his duties. His one defect was that he was morbidly sensitive to any slight, or even to any frank or merely light-hearted reference to him. It happened that one of his subordinates, a middle-aged man, married a young and inexperienced girl. The subordinate called with his wife on his chief, who happened to be a bachelor living with an unmarried sister. In the course of an animated conversation the young wife, apparently overwhelmed by her new happiness, remarked: "You two, of course, do not know what real family life means." Her unguarded statement was received with calmness and apparent assent.

Soon after this the subordinate made an application for promotion. As a married man, with the prospect of soon having a family, it was of importance to him to get an increase of salary. As a matter of routine the application was referred back to his chief for his opinion, and this man calmly but definitely refused to recommend the promotion. He did so again, two or three times, when further applications were referred to him. We do not know exactly what reason he gave; at that time general thinking was less democratic, and chiefs felt under no obligation to give any account to their subordinates of their likes and dislikes. We only know that the sister once told a friend of hers, also a patient of mine: "My brother cannot stand Mr. X. He simply cannot stand the man and his stupid wife."

I repeat: No walk of life is immune from opportunities of interference with the lives of others in a way, or to a degree, that is not quite justifiable, and from ulterior, subjective motives which are never realized and never admitted.

5. It is futile, and not even justifiable, to blame anti-social people of the types we have described so far. They cannot help being as they are ; and they are even less to blame for being blind to their inner motives. Guilty is society, and the State, in leaving the necessary self-education and enlightenment to the uninitiated individual, because the means exist today by which much—very much—misfortune, frustration, and tragedy could be prevented, and much productive energy gained for communal advantage. In view alike of psycho-analytical experience and of observations in everyday life, it is not justifiable simply to assume that an individual who is an expert in the technical or administrative side of his occupation, is automatically fitted to deal with the essential interests of his fellowmen. Even less does political experience alone provide the necessary qualification for social leadership and executive power.

The ordinary legal point of view ascribes the sole and whole responsibility for actions to the individual. The person who harms his fellow-being is blamed as much as the other person who benefits his fellow-being receives approval and praise. But for the social psychologist there must exist a somewhat modified measure of responsibility. The criminal or the paranoid behaves in a way so different from what is expected of men because a non-rational mental force drives him to do so, and to disregard the dictates of common sense and of social ethics. And, indeed, everyone, when under the sway of passion or in a pathological mental state, easily disregards the normal measure of behaviour, and blindly follows the urge of a biased psychic motive. The conclusion from this fact is that the others, who *are* in possession of a well-balanced outlook and in full possession of their senses, are responsible for not prohibiting the undesirable behaviour of particular individuals.

Politicians breathing hatred and aggression, and administrators and officials of a deficient moral character, count implicitly on the inertia, the cowardice, and even the passive approval of those who will not firmly stand up for social decency, and who do not possess sufficient ethical energy to take up the fight against social transgressors. The individual who is possessed by passion and prejudice, or is of pathological character, *knows* more or less that he is being aggressive toward the others ; he would give in if energetically opposed, because he would find it quite intelligible that his undutiful conduct or his aggression should be disapproved and not tolerated. He consequently takes the 'non-intervention' of the others as tacit approval of his neglect of duty or his aggression. *He* is unable to curb himself, since he has not the proper frame of mind for doing so. The main practical responsibility for any kind of hatred or social or administrative impropriety rests unquestionably upon the majority of 'normals' and 'decent' people. This is a clear postulate of up-to-date common sense; and there cannot be any substantial improvement of social conditions without the acceptance of the validity of this principle.

CHAPTER VI

CHILDREN AND PARENTS

1. The relationship of children to parents and of parents to children, the position, indeed, of a child amid the environment of adults in general, is a very complicate one; far more so than is realized by most people. This was certainly not adequately recognized in past centuries. It may safely be said that the first difficult situation which man has to face in his life is his presence, as a weak, immature, dependent creature, in the world of adults. And the effects of this highly differentiated condition are felt by a great number of people to the end of their days. They remain mentally, in various degrees, dependent—and resentful—children of their parents.

It has been the usual conception of parents that children are to be cared for, helped and guided, and also loved; and that on their part they have to obey, to give in, to adapt themselves to the wishes and habits of the adults. It has also been believed that all the difficulties that crop up in the course of family life are just abnormal and avoidable incidents, and their occurrence a nuisance and a misfortune. It is only peculiar that such 'incidental' deviations from the smooth programme of family life are of constant occurrence and occupy so large a place in the lives of parents and children.

We have to mark, learn, and inwardly digest the fact that no plan for the improvement of life, whether private or social, can fully succeed unless regard is had for the complex nature of man; and in particular for the complexity of what occurs in the mind of a growing child, and in its parents' minds, as a result of the mutual reaction between child and parents.

2. From the very start of its life, the infant is undergoing education through a combination of a granting attitude on the one hand and a restricting, regulating interference on the other. Wood or stone, when it is being moulded, also offers resistance ; anything in the nature of a creative alteration implies the overcoming of a measure of resistance to change. But wood and stone do not react ; that is, they do not develop new qualities in response to the interference. The infant, however, does so. It is easy to understand why. Consider, for instance, his bouts of hunger, appearing with not quite the regularity the parents would like. The inner, spontaneous rhythm of the infant's hunger is different from that which has come to mean regularity to the adults. In the progress of training, this apparently irregular rhythm, which is, perhaps, regular for the child, has to give way in favour of the artificial, the socially approved adult rhythm. There has to be brought into operation, within the child's physiological organization, a new clockwork which represses step by step the emergence of the hunger-feeling during the intervals which, according to the time-table of the adults, ought to be periods of rest. That means the creation of a new physiological 'instrument'.

But there is probably more in it than this. These regulative endeavours of the parents are bound to be felt by the infant at first as unpleasant compulsions, evoking resentment and the kind of reaction which later, in the progress to maturity, appears as hatred, resulting in some sort of spiteful behaviour.

No doubt the infant has an innate ability to develop his faculties of adaptation ; as a member of the human species he is destined to attain all the objectives of 'civilizing' restriction. But the process that leads to this final outcome has to overcome a continuous resistance against adaptation. The creation of new intra-psychic instruments is necessary to cope with that task and to overcome the unpleasantness, the pangs, of change. It must be realized that the various requirements of life necessitate a great variety and frequency of such events within the mind, in the service of adaptation.

3. We know for certain that a good many incidents of the educational compulsion in early life leave their marks ; this is clearly

indicated by the fact that the memory of them is retained. I do not believe that the recollection of the unpleasant and the difficult is simply a passive process, an inability to remove the pressure-marks of past life from the mind. We have rather to assume that the overcoming of any difficulty creates in fact, as explained above, a sort of new instrument of adaptation in the mind ; and that that which we experience as painful recollection is, at the same time, connected with the existence of such an adaptive ' counter-product ' within the mental organization. I do not suggest that such sequelae are always useful and beneficial. Much happens within the human mind that is not productive of harmony, pleasure, self-confidence, and mental strength.

If, in some emergency, a sensitive child has been given a fright, the memory of it will serve as a continual warning to avoid similar circumstances. Yet in most cases this warning is unnecessary for later life, since the same frightening incident may never occur again. But on many other occasions the recollection and the subsequently created inner ' counter-product ', which is experienced as warning and anxiety, does in fact serve a useful purpose. What we call experience in life is the sum of such accumulated counter-products, of recollections and intra-psychic warnings. Their sum-total enables man to behave in a more expedient, i.e. in an experienced, manner.

Those recollections of which the maintenance is more a nuisance than a source of improved behaviour are indicative of some disturbance in development ; that is to say, they signify a *neurotic* condition ; and if not removed from the psyche by subsequent pleasant experiences, they become a potential source of various neurotic breakdowns which may develop under the difficulties of later life. The ' infantile trauma ' [1] and the later ' recent conflict ' join hands in creating the full-blown neurosis of the adult.

We have dwelt on the description of this item, familiar to many people, in order to clear the way for the following discussion. We have to realize that the adaptive process, in its mental and physical aspects, goes along with continuous dramatic changes. Development through education implies intra-psychic struggle, i.e. complicated processes within the mind and nervous system. The more or less successful performance of all such necessary mental tasks manifests itself overtly as the average happiness of the child. This is very similar to what occurs within the complex digestive and assimilatory mechanism of man. A complexity

[1] ' Trauma ' means an attack on the integrity of body or mind.

of physio-chemical processes, thoroughly interwoven with the emotional life of man, takes place behind the screen of subjective awareness. Only disturbances of this process are realized as different illnesses, ranging from simple indigestion to the most difficult metabolic diseases ; otherwise the individual feels, in general, content and well. The individual, child or adult, *feels fairly well if the body and mind perform all their highly complicate tasks without his awareness, without too marked conscious knowledge of it on his part.*

Now, if it is realized how compound in their nature these things in fact are, the numerous incidents of disobedience, moodiness, spiteful behaviour, and even of aggressiveness bordering on criminality, must appear intelligible and more or less to be expected from the very start. They represent the inevitable occasional emergence of difficulties, which mostly are overcome intra-psychically,[1] but which remain latent. It is, therefore, rather by a special gift from nature that the child is not always naughty, and untidy, and difficult.

4. What makes all these inner complications remain as a rule underground and beyond detection is, however, not simply nature's automatism. The love and attention, the support and protection which the child enjoys from adults, the things that make up the 'social gain' within the family, render the whole regulative educational process easier. One definite factor in any successful relationship is the phenomenon of *identification.* There is an inborn tendency and faculty in man—in young and old alike—of identifying himself in different degrees with those in his environment whom he likes, appreciates, or admires.

Identification means the incorporation, as it were, of the image of a certain environmental person within oneself, making it part of oneself. Under favourable conditions the personality of every human being, living in any environment, incorporates during his life a number of these images ; and this process is essentially an enrichment of the mind and an increase of inner strength. It is easy to see that this identification or incorporation is very extensive and intensive in the case of relatives ; the emotional ties and the close community of living make for such a process. But it is equally true that the social environment of the individual gives ample opportunity of stimulating identifications with a great number of other persons.

[1] Within the mind, yet with no awareness.

Any person in one's environment who impresses one's mind by his personality, or by particular pleasant or forceful characteristics of his personality, initiates in the course of time this process of identification. The mind of the receiving individual, without ever being aware of it, incorporates that particular impression into the subconscious ; as if approving of and imitating some or all of the particular ways of that individual of his environment. It is clear that this identification is part and parcel of the other socially significant phenomenon called adaptation. It is the tendency to adaptation that finally brings about the identification, and the repeated attempts at identification with an ' environmental person ' facilitate in their turn the actual adaptation. We are able to adapt ourselves to another person's individuality if we are able to carry out a certain identification with him.

There are also, however, partial identifications which may imply that the mind not quite consciously identifies itself with certain qualities of another person, while consciously experiencing keen antagonism against the same individual. It is even certain that an individual may subconsciously identify himself, for instance, with his mother's primitive simplicity and at the same time consciously regret or despise that quality in his mother.

This identification, intensifying the positive sentimental ties of the child with his parents, cannot remain a smooth and simple process. Any occasion of conflict, of difference in interest between child and parent, in other words, any restrictive and controlling educational measure, brings into the foreground the child's awareness that he is separate and different from his parents and educators ; it throws into clear and painful relief the dissociated and even conflicting position in life of child and parent ; and this, naturally, is bound to interrupt or complicate the identification. At the moment of such a state of conflict the real, external parent or teacher, in virtue of his momentary strictness or insistence, contradicts the previously accepted image of his kinder self in the psyche of the child. This is not an easy condition for the child ; and its overcoming needs, almost on every occasion, a special intra-mental straightening-out process.

In the course of time, however, a great number of restrictive educational and ethical principles are accepted into the psyche of the child ; the latter is able to incorporate into himself the image of his parents at a time in the past when they seemed to him to be strict and intolerant ; provided that the task allotted to the child is not made too difficult or too wearying, and provided that the inborn psycho-nervous apparatus of the particular child is of average normality. This latter implies a fair capacity of adaptation, of accepting the new and gradually overcoming intra-psychic resistance and conscious resentment.

5. The educational implications of these facts are enormous, both for the intimate family circle and for the wider social community organized within the State. The requirements of our modern society with regard to the personal accomplishments of the individual are extensive and exacting. He is expected to be independent in thinking and poise, and at the same time to be considerate and susceptible to influence and suggestion ; selfish in one respect and altruistic in many others ; sufficiently trained to be able to grasp our complex social and scientific standards and yet not too sophisticated to be able to enjoy simple things and to display a natural naiveté.

Clearly, if the mental development of a particular child is not being systematically helped along, and if he is not being saved from superfluous intra-psychic effort ; if authority is being exerted in matters not really essential for later life, and if, on the other hand, educational insistence is neglected in matters of necessary discipline and training ; if school and family and society cannot conform, cannot supplement each other in influencing the child, then the daily task of inner adaptation in the mind of the child will not be as efficiently performed as it might be.

Clearly, a more helpful and more understanding attitude in the course of education can substantially ease the difficult tasks which the child's psycho-nervous system has to accomplish—the tasks involved in the free unfolding of his personality, both in the intellectual and in the emotional sphere. A modern education, based on thorough knowledge of all the processes it calls into play, is able to create an efficient and fairly happy individual, where the traditional methods of education might have resulted in the development of a personality far below the average requirements of life.

6. Let us now deal with the other side of the problem, the parents. Who are these parents, so much discussed today and held responsible for so much blessing and evil ? Are they not themselves weak mortals, fully occupied by their work, by money-making, engaged in the difficulties of social adaptation, called

upon to carry the burdens of citizenship, and, amid all this, facing the problems of their married status, of their love and sexual life?

Most of the parents are nothing but products of their own childhood, and of our existing mode of social life; they are, indeed, incapable of being better and more efficient educators and protectors of their children.

Any kind of activity needs energy; and parentage like any other. True, there is a gift from Nature, the parental instinct, with all the multiform interest in the child, love for it, the inclination to identify oneself with one's child, to sense its needs; and to do so during the different stages of development in which these needs are so different, and through which the parent grows mentally with his child: Nature has endowed man with the happiness and satisfaction, deep beyond words, that accompany the carrying out of his parental duties.

But man's effective energy is limited. The mind has immense creative potentialities. Yet in bearing burdens and troubles, in restricting one's own needs for pleasure and diversion, there are certain limits in going beyond which the parent may become irritable, moody, unjust, and altogether unfit to be a help to his child in the difficult task of intra-psychic adaptation described above.

And there is, unfortunately, more than this to be said. Only a small number of individuals have a tolerable faculty of adaptation for the married state, and similarly for finding sufficient sexual interest and higher emotional satisfaction in their partner for life. In most cases there ensues a gradual deterioration of the whole erotic-emotional function. The man and woman may feel that 'such things' are no longer of any great interest to them; they may even, for some people, appear burdensome and 'messy', as some of my woman patients have put it.

7. I may refer the reader to the later chapters on sexuality and on *unsuccessful repression*. This latter occurs, not in all, but in a good many cases, where the individual appears to have no interest in the sexual life. If man or wife suffers from unsuccessful repression, then, psychologically speaking, it is not true that the sexual urge has disappeared[1]; the term implies a state in which there is a constant drain on energy; and much irritability against children, strictness, hysterical moodiness of different kinds follow as the inevitable consequences.

[1] Cf. Ch. IX (7), p. 51.

Be it noted that children are not only a physical burden for the unhappy individuals who are not in possession of the full amount of their natural energy; they are, in particular, a constant reminder of sexuality. That is very significant; for many a neurotic individual finds his children merely a burden and a source of trouble, because the children are the products of a casual sexual act and of one which was not followed by a well-developed, harmonious love-relationship between husband and wife. "I have only the burden without its pleasures." So, though over-simplified, their neurotic formula might run. They will not be conscious that this is their feeling 'deep down', but the formula certainly expresses at least part of their mental disharmony.

Hatred against the conjugal partner, entirely repressed into subconsciousness, or at least suppressed as regards its overt manifestations, may make a father or mother irritable with the children. The usual transfer of sentiments from the original object to the substitute! But children of unhappy marriages are not only substitutes ready to hand as victims for attacks of irritability; they are part of the family bond, of the family bondage. And children occasionally, of course, make themselves a nuisance. More so, perhaps, under the above conditions than with married couples of better mental balance; since the parents' dissatisfaction extends to their children, and destroys a great deal of the children's natural spontaneity and gaiety.

Through the process of identification, children may feel too much of the disharmony of their parents; they try to find out who is the guilty one and who is the victim. Naturally, their mind is torn between the two parents. They feel affection for both, pity for both, resentment against both; and this complicated process has no end, no solution. Some children become neurotic and remain so throughout their lifetime, even after the parents have long died. The image of the parents is a more or less substantial part of the individual's intra-psychic structure; and it is a source of constant uneasiness to carry within the psyche the lifelong picture of ill-assorted parents.

The traces of an obviously unhappy marriage may be followed by an unsatisfactory development of the sexual faculty in the offspring. Marriage implies sexuality, and sexuality is potentially marriage—and for such children, implicitly, unsuccessful marriage. This link of ideas causes the subconsciousness to repress the sexual faculty, in order to safeguard the adolescent and the maturing boy and girl from marriage. A not infrequent 'complex', contributing to frigidity and erective impotency.

It is even enough mental trauma for a child when the balance of power in the family is too obviously shifted toward one side; if the father or the mother rules too obviously, whether by force or by means of blackmailing the conjugal partner into submission by nervous, restless, sulky, over-sensitive behaviour.

It should be briefly mentioned here that unsatisfied mothers, or women suffering from neurotic under-development of their sexual faculty, may pour out all their emotional interest over their children, and so unduly intensify the bonds of natural infantile fixation in them; thus obstructing the free path of their children to mental independence and fitness for their own later love-life.

The social organization could do much toward the improvement of family conditions: by lifting many anxieties from parents' shoulders, by providing more and better children's guidance clinics, and by improving the psychological conditions of married life in general. Let everyone have enlightenment on this matter; let the masses of docile people be relieved of the pressure of too much convention, of unnecessary shyness in these matters. And it is a grave social omission to leave a boy and girl alone in hours of perplexity, when they think that they are bound to marry but have justified doubts about the success of this step.

But it appears to the present author a social crime to leave unassisted in their helpless ignorance the young mothers who are faced for the first time with the greatest difficulties in human life—who find themselves disappointed in marriage, and left to contend, unaided and unadvised, with the burden of a household and with a husband lacking in the spirit and practice of a loving collaboration; and who under such conditions have later to bring up a more or less difficult or ailing infant.

The claims of duty, the conventional claims of social morals, are only an incentive to the continual expenditure of nervous energy required by such unfortunate conditions, but they cannot themselves provide that energy. Let us organize a society that offers the utmost support, at the start of their family life, to the considerable number of unhappy or constitutionally frail personalities. Much of the familiar neurotic or socially inferior character-traits which develop mainly in response to overstressed claims on the minds and bodies of half-mature young parents, and above all of the many 'girl-wives', might then disappear entirely.

The married state can become a source of increased social maturity, an incentive to increased understanding of social order and social collaboration. But in fact it becomes for so many couples the soil of neurotic attitudes, which restrict the development of the social sense, of higher love and general altruism. It must emphatically be declared that very much could be mended by an improved education of the population.

8. It is hardly possible to express in statistical figures the general social significance of difficult child-parent relationships. The material of the psycho-analyst, and that of the social worker, is naturally limited to those persons of various classes who seek the expert's help. But there are many who, from a natural sense of independence—and reserve or shyness—try to get over their difficulties by a mixture of yielding, neurotic responses, and aggressive attitudes ; in brief, by all the available mechanisms of human reactions and adaptation. We have in mind here solely the unsuccessful efforts at adaptation, not those of the persons, fortunately fairly numerous, who do possess the necessary mental capacity for coping in a more or less healthy way with family life.

If one is content to judge from the information gained from fairly intimate contact [1] with a hundred ‘ normal ’ families of the average type, the present author would be inclined to put the proportion of families with adequate mutual adaptation at one-third ; whilst about two-thirds have developed, quite obviously for the analyst, reactive [2] traits of a pathological or anti-social type under the burdens of existence, marriage, and the bringing-up of children. It appears to the author that about one-half of this latter group—parents and children alike—could have developed into more cheerful, less solitary, and less self-centred personalities if the social conditions had been more helpful. In about one-third of all cases there appears to be so much inherited peculiarity that no easy restoration of normality seems likely to be attainable.

CHAPTER VII

MARRIAGE

THERE is not the slightest doubt that the monogamic relationship between man and wife is the best attainable form of co-existence

[1] The author practised at one time as a physician.

[2] See p. 23 as to the meaning of ‘ react ’ and ‘ reactive ’. Cf. Ch. XI (5), p. 65.

of the two sexes, the form best suited to develop the deepest, richest, and most enduring emotional ties that can exist between two people who are not neurotic. This is so in principle, although there are so many marriages in which it is far from being so in fact. The one essential condition is that the partners are not neurotics—and this condition is not very frequently present. (A 'neurotic character' denotes a condition through which the individual is unable to cope with his emotional problems, or control the multitude of environmental influences, without mental stress and consequent disturbance of mental balance.)

Naturally, everybody is liable to be more or less neurotic at times. The essential point is that most of the difficulties in marriage are of a neurotic character. They are concerned, that is to say, with deficiencies in the faculty of mutual adaptation; with conscious or subconscious fixation [1] toward parents, brothers, sisters; with the survival of a primitive insistence upon personal prestige in marriage; and, of no less importance, with the lack of a healthy sexuality in both partners from the very start, owing to neurotic inhibitions or to an ingrained prejudice that looks upon sexuality as degrading or injurious to physical health. Where none of these undesirable conditions are seriously present, and where neither of the parties is paranoid (everywhere sensing slight and persecution), there can hardly be an unsuccessful marriage; though there may be difficult moments.

The overwhelming majority of unsuccessful marriages, judging from the author's analytical experiences, is caused by the fixation of one or both partners to their emotional past. People do not realize how much, in their subconsciousness, they retain and cherish the picture of their nearest relatives and consider them, or people like them, as the ideal of a partner-for-life. This may be so although they have no conscious sense of such a preservation of their emotional past. They seem to be entirely unaware of this fixation. But generally, when undergoing analysis, they clearly betray some knowledge of this fixation. Many a man contrasts the breakfast his up-to-date wife prepares for him with the meals he used to receive from his simple but loving and self-sacrificing mother. Many a man wants his wife to be fashionable and not a family slave, and yet, at bottom, he is full of admiration for the ways of his mother, who slaved away early and late and had no other interest than the children. Many

[1] 'Fixation' denotes an attachment, usually to near relatives, which substantially interferes with the faculty of loving others who are strangers. It is regarded as a 'halt' in mental development, a 'psycho-sexual infantilism'.

a man thinks that his sister is nicer, more attractive, or a more reliable character than his wife—and so on, with infinite variations, and in men and women alike.

It can, apparently, do a great deal of harm to the modern man and woman of developing individuality, to be tied to their family past, to take for granted the superiority of their parents over all other human beings. An ingrained belief of this sort is hardly compatible with good adaptation in marriage. For the partner, naturally, is always different in type, is an individual.

CHAPTER VIII

THE EMOTIONS OF MAN

1. IMAGINE yourself in a condition of satisfactory relaxation, after a good night's sleep, in good physical health and with no worries or difficult problems breaking into the harmonious level of your feeling ; *you experience the whole of your self, body and mind together ; you perceive your psycho-somatic organization, by feeling.* This psychological structure I propose to call the *affect-ego*, because it is one's self, but experienced less by intellectual apperception than by feeling. All the specifically coloured emotional states—anger, fear, tense expectation, or the tension through suspicion, and similarly the various shades of pleasure, of contentedness, of thrill and joy—*all these specific emotional conditions are only modifications of that fundamental affect-ego.* In topography we conceive peak and valley as modifications of the horizontal plain ; and similarly it may be suggested that the particular emotions—the peaks and valleys—should be conceived as variations of that basic affect-ego.

If we had not that fundamental feeling of our self, we should not be able to experience the various emotions. There is, indeed, a condition known to the psychiatrist as depression and melancholia (not quite the same thing as what we call in ordinary life ' being depressed '), in which this feeling of the self is disturbed. A patient in this condition feels himself substantially altered, incapable of clear thinking, feeling, and enjoying. With the disturbance of his self, of his affect-ego, is closely connected a more or less substantial disturbance of his faculty of experiencing the other specific emotions, sorrow, fear, love, and merriment, as they actually exist.

2. Let us keep in mind this aspect of our self, this perception of one's self by feeling ; it is, I believe, the personality-factor of most importance to the social life of the individual.

The environment, animate and inanimate, is being experienced in so far as it alters this homogeneous affect-ego. True, the environment, physical and social alike, seems to affect partly our body and partly our mind—as it were, in separate kinds of attack. For instance, cold or hunger, or a knock, hurts and brings physical discomfort to the body, whereas financial worries, or threats to our social position, or to our happiness, trouble the mind. But, in fact, that part which ultimately feels and suffers all the various attacks is the *unity of the above affect-ego*. And it is the same *affect-self* in its unity that enjoys the enjoyable.

Any exploiting pressure of the potent environment on the weak wage-earning individual hurts and breaks down this *affect-ego* ; and any institution of a socially beneficent character, including the measures and means of general security, average peace, and stability of conditions—all this supports and keeps well the affect-ego of people. The affect-ego is the ' extract ' of body and mind through which a person feels himself—the personality-factor that ' feels ' happy or unhappy, that ' feels ' well or unwell in the case of good-health or ill-health. It is generally acknowledged today in medicine that, in any physical illness, apart from the feeling of specific complaints, there is an individually coloured mental experiencing of the condition of ill-health in general.

Any social condition that imposes unnecessary pressure and restriction on people attacks their affect-ego. Any social condition that robs the individual of his sense of security hurts his affect-ego. I suggest, on the other hand, that the affect-ego is also the core of the social personality, it is that that determines the quality of the good or bad citizen, the good or bad fellow-being. The more satisfactory, the more level are the emotion-egos of individuals, the more do genuine peace and genuine happiness fill the spheres of communal life. And all the disharmony of our day, the restlessness and dissatisfaction, the disunity and universal tendency toward animosity and the struggle of all against all, the insincerity even where there is no special advantage in being insincere, the nervous sham-peace in social life—all this is due to the fact that the emotion-egos of people are under constant strain, owing to complicated conditions of living, and to the experience of injustice and enslavement. The person with a harmonious affect-ego reacts—that is to say, lives and acts—in an essentially harmonious way, in a more or less logical way ; he becomes insincere and aggressive only when real conditions require this self-defence. But when the affect-ego is stirred up, when the personality is continually 'kept under', and body and mind are suffering from strain, some sort of neurotic behaviour of the individual is bound to ensue.

3. People are not yet aware of the physiological significance of man's emotional life. They think only of the particular emotions that accompany special occasions, experiences and actions of man. This, I think, is a mistake, and a very one-sided view. There is no moment of human life, whether in waking or sleeping, not a single action of our organs, no part of any physiological process occurring within our self, that is not closely accompanied by emotional changes. Only, these are inarticulate, 'silent' emotions.[1] They are emotions that are not recognizable unless observed with special attention. Observe yourself whilst eating, dozing, quietly playing, or experiencing and acting in any way at all—none of this happens without a simultaneous process of some kind of feeling. Human life cannot go on without continuous emotional life ; and, in fact, this continuous emotional energy is probably indispensable for normal life.

The functioning of our stomach and bowels, the respiration and blood circulation and all the natural processes, create as much emotional experience as does any mental activity. And the sum-total of the emotions emanating continuously from all over the organism makes up the affect-self above.

4. Sufficient and appropriate food, with all the necessary vitamins ; sunshine and air ; hygienic and fairly comfortable housing ; public transport saving as much energy as possible, with frequent services in all directions and pleasant, well-upholstered coaches ; not much noise on the streets, no industrial fumes and poisonous products in residential districts ; green parks and benches wherever possible ; public lavatories in far greater number than has been usual hitherto, and for men and women alike—all these factors, if provided satisfactorily, would contribute to a better development and better-preserved integrity

[1] We speak in neurology of 'silent regions' of the brain, parts whose damage does not create crudely manifest symptoms and whose normal role may therefore not be appreciated, but the activity of which is nevertheless continually in process. I suggest a similar expression for the affect.

of the affect-ego ; and the deficiencies in all these fields of existence are continuous attacks on the emotions of man.[1]

The lack of appreciation of the beauties of Nature, art, and literature, and the less refined sensual life (sexual and palatal pleasures), in the great majority of working-class people, are largely due to the pressure of economic insecurity, but no less so to the enslavement of mind and body by the expenditure of so much energy on hurrying, queueing, and travelling in crowded and unpleasant public conveyances. In their home life, too, the many and various inconveniences and shortcomings constitute continual attacks on the emotional spheres. The mind has to acquire indifference to such concrete deficiencies, in order to be hardened to this low standard of living. But with this goes under-development or even deterioration of the higher emotional spheres.

In another group of people, who do still possess sensitiveness to emotional and sensual experience, the above-mentioned deficiencies of daily life constitute, as suggested, a source of repeated attacks on their emotion-self ; and they definitely reduce the capacity of such individuals to be fairly harmonious, and socially pleasant and useful members of humanity.

The first-mentioned group, as a rule, do not manifestly display the deficient structure of their emotional self. Their subjective feeling of their self appears not to be disturbed—but only so long as conditions of social order and external force are operative. The tragic and uncontrollable events, however, that emerge in times of revolutionary change are proof enough of the deficient emotional make-up of ' the masses '. Their apparent indifference and lack of sensitiveness in ordinary times does not prevent the manifestation of unbridled cruelty in extraordinary periods of history.

Inner freedom and spontaneity, and relaxation in the measure necessary for well-being, depends not only on one's inborn capabilities, not only on appropriate impressions received in one's youth, but on the sum-total of the above lifelong environmental influences ; and each separate item of them is contributory to the individual's affect-ego. Yet, as has been said, the quality of the affect-ego largely determines whether or not the particular individual can behave calmly under average conditions without undue excitement, and whether or not the individual has the desirable nervous energy, enabling him to be as good and kind and loving, as dutiful and tolerant as he is expected to be, and as he himself would naturally like to be.

[1] Cf. also Ch. XIII (3), p. 77, and Ch. XXIV (1), p. 137.

It appears as if man actually has a certain amount of free will; as if he is able, in a limited degree, to decide upon his ethical behaviour. Yet one must emphatically point out, what is well known to any observant psychiatrist—if he is not very prejudiced in favour of certain ideologies—that *the ease and the steadiness in carrying out the dictates of logic, insight, duty, and good intentions, is largely dependent on the given conditions.* The quality of the *affect-ego*, which is the result of different mental, physical, and environmental conditions, finally decides, I think, on this point.

5. I think the average man does not receive enough beauty to maintain the emotional balance of his personality. The enjoyment of products of art, if made a regular habit, can fill many gaps in individual satisfaction. The usual type of popular wireless programme merely fills up the time, and does little if anything to satisfy that psychological need. Disharmonies within the mind, and dissatisfaction due to an insufficient measure of the deeper joy that meets the soul's need, constitute universal human fate. The philosophers of past centuries had great faith in the refining effect of suffering and self-denial ; moralists even praised the existence of pain and disappointment as necessary for calling forth the higher human virtues.

Conditions must have changed considerably. There is hardly a human being today who does not, during his youth and early manhood, discover ample sources for that necessary amount of disappointment. Many a reader of this volume will be only too ready to agree that, if the conditions here described are factual conditions of universal validity, then, in the old phrase, life is hard. But—that is our modern belief—to a substantial extent it is needlessly so. In past centuries it was not so clearly realized that human suffering can and therefore should be substantially diminished ; that the great masses of people can and therefore should participate in the blessings of social improvements.

We need much less, then, of the philosophy of suffering, and much more of the enjoyment of the higher arts. Public galleries and occasional lectures on art are not enough. People are too tired to leave home and regularly visit such places. The forty-hour week, with two days left for family life and the regular cultivation of the higher arts, constitutes one of the minimal social requirements. But beyond this, beauty must be brought home to man, must surround him where he lives and works. First of all, the pupils of secondary school age should be enabled and helped, more than they are at present, to enjoy and appreciate fine music and pictures. And, as far as possible, the method of *free, 'intuitive' drawing and colouring should also be employed.*[1] That means that the child should be encouraged to draw forms and to colour them, simply following his momentary inspiration, without striving after the representation of any real object. All this, and more than this, should be an indispensable part of education. *So much so, that the grown-up youth, the young adult, should feel his craving for art, for relaxation through art, to be a basic mental necessity,* and not merely an occasional luxury.

The number of individuals who would benefit greatly from such reformed education should not be under-estimated. Even without knowing much about the particular psychological significance of art and beauty, there is a general realization of the refining emotional influence of such interests. But the fact can be accounted for by a scientific theory. This leads us to the much discussed topic of *Sublimation.*[2]

6. Clearly there exists a transformation, i.e. a *sublimation*, of the sexual urge with physical aims into the refined emotional attitude of love, appreciation, and adoration of the beloved partner. The degree of this transformation is, as is well known, individually variable ; it can, in some people, and under particular conditions of life, be very considerable. Yet in this instance the transformation obviously occurs within the spheres of the same instinct, and its peripheral, complementary fields. Emotional attachment, biased appreciation, the realization of attractive qualities not recognized by strangers, tenderness and increased care for each other's well-being,[3] are closely combined attitudes in the relationship between members of the opposite sexes ; the shifting of the emphasis toward the mere psychic factors is quite obvious, and this type of sublimation is easy to understand.

As to the apparent sublimation of sex into other, heterogeneous[4] tendencies, such as religion, sport, social activities of different kinds, scientific research, and so on, the difficulty of understanding such transformation of libidinal interests, and even of energies appertaining to the sphere of sex, as stated by Freud, has always been great. The present author would like to advance—though

[1] Cf. Herbert Read, *Education through Art*, 1943.

[2] See J. C. Flugel, *Sublimation*, in the Br. J. Ed. Psych., 1942.

[3] According to McDougall, the tenderness-factor in the love-relationship comes not from the sexual but from the parental instinct.

[4] That is, non-sexual manifestations.

only sketchily—the following modification of the usual conception of this problem. He would first refer the reader to the explanations already given of the homogeneous feeling of our ' self '. It was stated that the sum-total of the self-perception of the physiological and mental processes occurring within the human organization constitutes the foundation of the affect-self. To put it now in different terms : I think the repercussions of all the processes occurring within the human organization—desires, repressions, and similar intra-psychic movements included—integrate into the unitary feeling of our living ' self '. In one or another sector of psycho-affective life, fluctuations and crises always take place ; but, within a certain limit, the self-feeling as a whole is not affected by this.[1] *It is as if there were a mutual compensation within the individual spheres of the totality of emotional processes.*

It appears to me that following a successful repression in one field—such as is necessary with sexuality or aggressiveness—there arises, as it were, an increased hunger in other spheres, an increased productive potentiality, *in order to satisfy and to maintain the balance of the affect-self.* An arbitrary kind of ' distracting one's attention ' cannot have the same sublimating effect as the compensatory rise of an intrinsic disposition, closely appertaining to the basic components of the affect-self of the individual concerned. The particular conditions and effective methods of sublimation of the sexual urge are, consequently, of a highly individual character. There must ensue a certain spontaneous thirst or readiness for a particular sphere of creative activity. And this particular substituting interest must be fitted to restore the balance of individual conditions that results in a satisfactory feeling of the self.

Here we have to consider the factor of fashionableness. People are readily inclined to like, and to enjoy, things which are generally approved or are in vogue. This does not merely indicate a meek yielding, resulting from lack of individuality. The sharing of the aims, desires, activities, and enjoyments of the majority, and particularly of the ' higher circles ' acknowledged as such by the majority, can make this liking genuine. And we may accordingly assume that the satisfaction of the ' social instinct ', through following in the generally approved taste of one's social environment, is in itself a factor which may contribute to the emotional balance ; and which may help in the process of a successful, satisfying sublimation. This factor of enjoying in community with others is a well-known element in the increase

[1] There is a mental ' homeostasis '.

of human pleasure. Taking our meals, listening to music or theatrical performances, or attending lectures or sporting events, normally brings a more intense enjoyment in the company of others than in solitude.

And similarly, the awareness of being one of those following a certain fashion, contains a substantial factor of subjective satisfaction ; in my view, a satisfaction of the ‘ social instinct ’.

Since, on this view, the particular pattern of a person’s desires and satisfactions depends, to a certain degree, on the moulding social process, it is obvious that communal organization could do much for the success of the process of sublimation. The first thing needed is a careful and comprehensive study, free from the customary psycho-analytical one-sidedness ; and also free from the traditional simplicity that assumes that any kind of substitute is expedient, and that any amount of suppression of instincts is possible, ‘ given only the will ’.

7. In individual therapeutic practice it is easy to advise one’s patients on the helpful possibilities of sublimation open to them. But there is an urgent need for broader social studies, for consideration of the particular mental make-up of the different occupational strata, their particular difficulties, and the possible satisfactions connected with their particular field of activity, and for then considering the possibilities of supplementing their particular life with additional individual modes of satisfaction.

It is, of course, perfectly possible to break down the personality of an individual while still retaining his physical abilities, and thus reducing him for a number of years to an automaton, working for the benefit and satisfaction of others. But that does not solve the *problem of successful and creative sublimation.* For this there must be a certain integrity of the psycho-somatic personality, and a *biological capacity to sublimate.* Much depends on the freedom of the inner personality of the individual, on his genuine approval of his intimate and wider environment, for the sake of which repression and sublimation of instinctual tendencies has to take place. Much depends on the valuation of art, science, religion, and sport by the sublimating individual. Above all, much depends on the amount of satisfaction in other fields of mental life, if the individual is to be able to bear the efforts of repression and to succeed in the sublimation of his sexual and aggressive tendencies. The more satisfactory is the intra-psychic relation of the individual to his family problems, and to the social organization, and the less burdened he is by avoidable, unnecessary denials and pressures, the better, as a rule, must be his capacity for a productive, and also for a subjectively satisfying, sublimation of sex and aggressiveness.

8. Experience shows that a person whose sense of beauty and art has been developed at an early age, so becoming an intrinsic part of his mind, may observe the lack of harmony and proportion in the existing world more frequently, and may feel it more keenly, than most people ; but it is equally true that he is at the same time *better fitted to cope with the shocks of denial and social pressure. This means that he possesses an effective means of sublimation and compensation.* Perhaps that is so because even the passive enjoyment of art—whether music, painting, literature, or acting—goes along with a more or less active creation within the mind. The person experiencing the artistic work and performance of others, by the process of identification and intra-psychic interpretation, feels, as it were, the production of it in himself.

But there is also, I should imagine, a further explanation of this powerful effect of substitution through art for repressed tendencies or denied experiences. Though the particular sources of satisfaction are numerous—physical and mental occurrences of great variety—their contribution to the subjective structure of self-feeling may, I think, be more or less of a similar kind. If I may describe this conception in a rather venturesome way, I should like to put it thus : Every process connected with satisfaction consists of three elements. The first is that of the process in its objectivity. Then there is the accompanying emotional experience. In the satisfaction of hunger and appetite, and similarly in the erotic spheres, this double aspect of the experience is clear. I refer to the well-known conception of McDougall, who taught that emotions are the subjectively experienced aspects of the instinctual striving and action. We can now imagine an additional factor. From the specifically coloured emotional experience of a satisfying action there splits off, as it were, *a contribution to the general sense of well-being*, i.e. a contribution to that feeling which I have called the *affect-self*. The same double aspect, but within the spheres of subjective experience, is imaginable in mental processes—in seeing and thinking : there is first *the particular sensory or intellectual experience, and in addition there is its contribution to the affect-self.*[1]

[1] Compare the idea of ' general emotionality ' or the ' e ' factor suggested by Burt.

If this conception be acceptable—and there is much more to be said in its favour—the substitution of one tendency by another becomes more intelligible ; since there is *a mutual supplementation by similar—or at least not entirely heterogeneous—elements of experiencing. And probably the enjoyment of art contains this general subjective factor in a greater measure ; thus enabling the individual to carry out his substitutions and sublimations with the aid of this sphere to a substantial degree, and with substantial success.*

CHAPTER IX

SEXUALITY IN ITS CULTURAL AND SOCIAL ASPECT

1. The number of publications during the last forty years on the psychology and the social aspect of the spheres of sex is very large and hardly possible to survey. Many of these, though not the majority, are really good ; and they have made a considerable contribution to enlightenment and have led to some practical improvement. But a brief statement of our knowledge of the subject, and, to begin with, of its social aspect, may give the reader some additional insight into its problems. In any case, it is necessary to include the subject in a work such as the present one.

Limitations and regulations of sexual life and sexual feeling have been the main characteristic and buttress of every civilization based on the biblical or almost any other religious conception. Even beyond the range of religious ideologies, certain rites regulating sexual relations were peculiar to many primitive cultures.[1] The realization of their necessity, or rather of the particular character of this biological urge, appears to be as old as human history. We are concerned here, however, with this sphere of life as a problem for our present civilization.

There will never, in any imaginable future, be any cultural standard that will dispense with the conception of sexual morality as unnecessary and unjustified. Humanity will never lose the conviction that sexuality is something particularly significant and full of complications. We shall always continue to surround it with special attention ; and we shall always struggle to diminish the 'polar tension' between its elementary urgency on the one hand and its relationship to the finer, higher life of love between

[1] Cf. Freud, *Totem and Taboo*, 1919.

man and woman on the other. And there will never be a complete solution for all the difficulties involved, both social and moral.

The growing individualism of man in general and the increasing emancipation of woman in particular have thrown up the difficulties of the problem in a tragic, appalling degree. In principle, we want to have the sexuality of man and woman closely bound up with personal love and mutual fidelity. As far as possible, we want to limit this mutual relationship to a condition of legalized marriage, with lifelong bonds. The safeguarding of the family, i.e. of the children, and the protection of the woman, who as she grows older becomes sexually less attractive to any stranger, absolutely justify such an aim, even from a utilitarian point of view. And the ideal of a woman devoted sexually, if possible, to one man only in her life —or, after failure with him, to another, but only by way of correcting an initial mistake—has so far essentially retained its supreme place in our emotionally coloured thinking, far more than in the case of the man.

The primitive jealousy of the possessive man, characteristic of the savage, continues into the refined desire of the present-day man to have a ' pure woman ' for himself. This fact, in the light of the other fact that most men have had sexual relations before marriage, or before falling seriously in love with somebody for their lifetime, constitutes an obvious injustice against the female sex. Yet we cannot help it.

2. There is, beyond question, a certain advantage for the man in having had sexual experience before getting married. In consequence of the necessary restriction of sexual manifestation by education in the early life of every human being, there is scarcely ever a normal, natural, spontaneity in the exercise of the erotic part of love-life. *Inhibitions of various kinds have been accumulated within the mind during the early and more advanced educational periods.*

A child is trained from infancy to regard his organs of evacuation as things that must be kept strictly hidden. And the universal tendency of infants and small children to play with these parts of their body is met with more or less energetic educational corrective measures, smacking of the hands being frequently employed to accompany the spoken expressions of horror. People do not realize the possible ill-effects of these painful measures on the later development of the individual. Their chief educational aim is, however, attained: there ensues in the psyche *an automatic linking up of the idea of 'private parts and sexual sphere' with that of 'socially more or less disapproved'.*

The subconscious recollections of the physical punishment or of its threat, connected with such infantile playing, may add the component of fear to this association of ideas.

Another and a very important source of anti-sexual inhibition originates in the following factor. From nature itself the curiosity of the child, directed toward observing the naked body of others, and especially of those of the opposite sex, does not exclude its nearest relatives, such as parents and brothers or sisters. On the contrary, these persons are, as a rule, the first ones actually available for the imagination of the child. And, similarly, when more or less intense sexual feelings begin to direct the interest of the growing child toward the opposite sex, it is again not nature's command to exclude near relatives. Only artificial educational influences bring about the repression of this erotic interest in the naked body and the sex-quality of near relatives.

And with this fact goes, more or less, a brake on the sexual tendencies. The influence of this incestuous repression extends more or less to sexuality in general. The subconscious mind at first cannot make a clear distinction between the relatives who have become sexual taboos and other people who are destined, in later life, to become the approved potential objects of the libidinal interest of the adult.

No doubt these early educational measures lay the foundation for the shyness and sense of self-restriction that enables the grown-up individual to comply with the broader sexual morals of his social environment; both in his actions and also in his particular ideology on this subject.

If, then, the adolescent and the young adult has to carry out over a considerable number of years a suppression of his sexual urge, this may be accompanied by a simultaneous deeper-reaching process. His mind, in a degree varying from individual to individual, represses the healthy idea of sexuality altogether, in order to save him from continuous displeasure or conflict. All this might still be very beneficial. But this condition may now revive the subconscious anti-sexual tendencies that were in operation during the years of earlier development. The recollection of the strict educational process aiming at the exclusion of near relatives from the sexual spheres; of the strict suppression of masturbation in the young by the educating adults; of the threats and deterrent and embarrassing utterances on this matter

—the recollection of all these influences may restore the past actuality of the fears and the intra-psychic fights they produced, and may overpower the *subconscious*, owing to the deficient counter-balance of mature sexual interests. It is intelligible that, if the scale of sexual maturity contains little or nothing of concrete experience, the other scale, representing the infantile past, may outweigh it.

Sexual neurasthenia of all kinds,[1] and of various degrees, may be the outcome. And though as a rule such a condition is easily curable, ignorance, or shyness, or a hypocritical attitude in these matters, prevent most people from seeking help at the start of their marriage and of its difficulties. But I have found that the financial burden connected with a psycho-analysis, and its duration, is the most frequent reason why people neglect this aspect of their lives, and disregard this potential enemy of their married state.

3. There will always be a desire—and a social and cultural need—to cultivate the idea of sexual continence maintained from ethical motives, insisting on the central position of love, and on the principle of monogamous marriage. We all realize the need for such an ideal in our cultural pattern. And yet it is necessary to point out, with the same emphasis, the practical impossibility, and even undesirability, of forcing young men to remain abstinent, at all costs, until their marriage—which may come late, very late, or even never. As for the absolute social pressure exerted, through contempt or even through moral or hygienic intimidation, on people who would not find happiness, and would feel no element of natural spontaneity, in enforced sexual abstinence, one is bound to find this still more unjustifiable. It has been explained, though only briefly, how the resulting condition of repressed sexual tension may lead not only to neurotic dysbalance, not only to intensification of subconscious anti-sexual inhibitions, which may harm the sexual faculty in later life ; but, what is more important, to marriages being entered into solely under the urge of suppressed sexuality, a course which, in many cases, may prove anything but desirable or likely to prove successful.

[1] Erective impotency, ejaculatio praecox, lack of libidinal feeling, etc. Such disturbances in the man's sexuality are of far greater significance for the success of marriage than the frigidity of the woman. The latter may at times spontaneously improve in the course of a satisfactory marriage-relationship, if the husband is in possession of the art of love. And even if this does not occur, a number of frigid women appear to tolerate their condition without manifest neurotic complaints.

Religious ideology claims absolutely : " So be it : morality is worthy of sacrifices." This is unquestionably true, in so far as it concerns principles of unquestionably universal and indispensable social ethics. The conditions of the actual world around us, however, do not confirm the absoluteness of the principle under discussion. It must be left, therefore, to religious denominations, and to other organizations for cultivating and advocating ethical principles, to keep up the idea of ' sexual continence at any cost '. On the other hand, it must be the absolute duty of the State, and of its higher educational institutions, to maintain the awareness of those concerned of the merely relative validity of what is, in itself, certainly a high spiritual principle—a principle that may well be considered actually an elementary human tendency, though with only a limited scope for materialization in practical life. The State must see to it that nobody shall be artificially subjected on this point to more mental conflicts than are necessary and endurable for him. In particular, young people, suggestible and susceptible to higher forms of idealism, and at the same time easily frightened into unworthy submission, should enjoy the protection of the State against the unscrupulous propaganda of the fanatic, ignorant or learned.

It is impossible to give any clear indication as to the permissible degree of public religious anti-sexual propaganda ; the topic itself, the inevitable bi-polarity [1] of our social interest in both aspects, will never permit a clear delineation. There will never be—and let us emphasize this—a final decision as to whether the religious, anti-sexual principle, or the free right of the individual to enjoy this sphere of his instinctual life, is the preferable, the ' only valid ' principle. Both appear indispensable ; and the preservation of a balance between the two trends will always remain a new and separate task for each individual. It is for the State, however, to safeguard the mental health and the working capacity of its citizens ; and this is certainly not done by thoughtless and biased intimidation and by the spreading of prejudiced or only theoretical principles.

Let the wider public understand that most young people, who very readily submit to the principle of the ' sinfulness and baseness of sexuality ', are potential neurotics in a psychological sense. There exist in their subconscious mind different effective motives (which we cannot detail here) that make the young susceptible to propaganda for ' purity ' ; not from a true sense for higher tendencies, but because subconscious neurotic factors in them

[1] Oscillating between two extreme points.

approve of the anti-sexual sentiment. One instance only : There is, as is well known, in certain individuals *an over-stressed emotional fixation to the mother or sister*; in others, there is a not quite conscious contempt for mother or sister and, by way of generalization, for the female sex as a whole. It is logical that such complexes in deeper spheres should readily 'join hands' with religious anti-sexual principles ; since this latter attitude helps to carry out the 'intentions' of the above complexes, i.e. to keep the man aloof from women in general, and especially from sexual association with them. The victory of the moralistic propaganda in such individuals reveals itself, accordingly, as little more than exploitation, in the cause of morality, of the 'weak' ; a phenomenon so frequent in all other spheres of social life, when sacrifices are required from people.

I recollect the case of a young man who once visited my consulting-room because of a tremor of his hand. It was obvious that he was suffering from the insidious condition called *post-encephalitis* (sleeping sickness). He was 25 years of age, and intellectually and emotionally fairly normal. He felt, and was, physically inferior to his fellows ; and he looked for spiritual comfort to attendance at the religious meetings of a mission. The leader of this mission encouraged him by saying that his tremor might be only 'functional', i.e. brought about by mental stress, and curable. At the same time he encouraged him to remain at any rate chaste, since this way of life would contribute to physical health, and also make him beloved by God. And now, he said, he would like to know whether his tremor was in fact only a psychogenic one. I could not commit the cruelty of telling him the clinical truth ; and answered in an evasive manner. Then he said : "You know, I am particularly interested in the matter of sexual activity. I have been told that continence will save much of my vital energy." On this point the answer of the neurologist was : "That is not quite true ; if you happened to be married already, nobody of a sane mind would warn you about evil consequences. But your question is a problem of religious conscience. Many a man of strict morality, ascetic deep down in his subconsciousness, and firmly believing in the sinfulness of sexual activity, is in danger if he does not take heed of this inner moral tendency of his mind, of experiencing actual physical discomfort after sexual activity ; this is due to the intense consequences of a mental conflict." And then came his admission : "I must confess to you, I have tried it and feel much relieved."

That is about all that I wish to say here as regards the male. And now a few remarks, brief but of importance, with regard to the female sex. No doubt there is no logical justification for taking up a different attitude toward the freedom of the female world in this sphere of life. Unquestionably, it is both right and expedient that the individual herself should decide this matter, according to the balance between her own tendencies toward sexual restraint before marriage and toward a more natural course.

4. And yet there is something more to be said. And this additional remark may apply also to some men. It is very noticeable in many women, if you analyse their dreams, and also their free associations during a more advanced stage of their psycho-analysis, that their first mature sexual experience, and notably the first actual intercourse, has left deep impressions behind in their conscious and subconscious spheres. And this, if later they marry someone else, may create difficulties in adaptation to their actual conditions of life ; though they remain unconscious of the source of their difficulty and irritability. Unquestionably a sexual experience means more to a woman's psyche than to a man's. This appears certain at least for the members of our civilization, so far as is shown by careful research. The artificial educational influences play, naturally, a great part in this ; the little girl, from the very start, is surrounded by the accepted, stricter claims on the woman's self-limiting morality in everything that concerns her body and the libidinal emotions. Yet it appears as if the female sex were, in fact, even by nature more susceptible to such a modifying influence of education. I am speaking, of course, of the average person ; whilst realizing that a minority of men can also be considered as feminine in this respect ; and, on the other hand, not a few women do not conspicuously reveal this monogamic type of subconscious attitude.

We know very well the probable historical background of this development. The man was physically the stronger, and was possessive and jealous. The woman was the weaker partner ; and besides, she was subject to the physiological restrictions connected with pregnancy and the ties of motherhood. Every woman is a potential mother, both physically and mentally. And no future civilization can dispense with the motherly and womanly tenderness, with the woman's bashfulness, or with the mother's superior devotion to her family. It will probably always be the case that the woman's sexual tendencies are more interwoven than the man's with the function of sublimating repression. This sexually inhibiting factor may remain operative in a particular female individual even if, from intellectual considerations, she wishes to disregard it. The ultimate effect of the conflict on mental harmony can never be estimated in advance. The conscientious psycho-analyst feels bound to point out the complicate nature of the facts.

Much as we must disapprove of the comparative subjection of the female sex, rendering the woman the passive object—and not infrequently the unhappy victim—of the particular personality and the intimate peculiarities of the man who chances to become her legal husband ; much as it may seem desirable that the woman, too, should have some preliminary experience of men of various kinds, in order to make her ultimate choice in more or less freedom and knowledge—it remains true that such preliminary sexual experiences may deeply encroach upon her psyche.

Nevertheless, our womenfolk ought to enjoy the same freedom of mind as men ; they should not be impelled by parents and schools to keep their feelings under unnecessarily rigid control, to subject them to undue repression. In brief, they should be allowed to enjoy unlimited freedom of mind and more spontaneity of feeling. As a result of this they will be in a far better, healthier position, far better able to keep watch on their *actions*, and to decide upon their course in life before marriage and in marriage ; and, if need be, to take with courage in due time, before it is too late, the necessary steps even for dissolving a formal tie which cannot be a blessing to either party, and can only be a source of nervous troubles for their children.

5. It can be definitely stated that the present-day man's fundamental desire is rather the libidinal [1] human relationship than the mere sexual act. Many individuals may seem to disprove the general validity of this assertion, but it can safely be stated that this is only due to external conditions of their life, and even more to their intra-psychic inhibitions, which do not permit the clear manifestation of this universal human desire for a refined love-relationship. There are people whose neurosis (subconscious

[1] 'Libidinal' is a psycho-analytical expression denoting any part-tendency in human love-life in a broader sense.

disharmony) results in such 'fear of love'. But the present author cannot remember a single individual whom he has had the opportunity to analyse who had not quite obviously this human desire of entering into emotional and spiritual relationship with his sexual partner. Everybody is potentially capable of falling in love—provided certain circumstances crop up, which stimulate in him the development of an emotional attachment to one particular member of the opposite sex. It may be a specific quality of the partner that appeals to the subconscious requirements of the particular individual. Or it may be an exceptional condition of his own mind due to subconscious processes at work in him at that period which make him suddenly feel deeper love toward somebody; though such an emergence of love may be quite unexpected to himself. But the fact that such a socially refined desire for love does exist in everybody cannot be denied. And it seems really not impossible, by improved cultural and social conditions, to enable more and more individuals to overcome their 'love-inhibitions' and to strive for this refined form of sexual relationship.

6. It is generally advisable for the individual to try to adapt himself mentally to the stricter rather than to the laxer moral conceptions on sexual behaviour obtaining in the particular country, or the particular social stratum, in which he lives. It is not justifiable to try to persuade people to defy their conscience. This was the attitude of the late Dr. Stekel, one of the greatest experts on the psychology of sex. And I personally feel that the same applies, in the absence of pressing reasons, to defiance of the conventional attitude of one's social environment. The loss in self-confidence and in social spontaneity may be greater than the gain in relieving the pressure of temporary continency.

Yet if, at any time, a person who is free of the mutual obligations of marriage, after examining his own case carefully, finds that the maintenance of the usual sexual morals means to him nothing more than an undesirable frustration, the source only of unpleasant repression without any spiritual satisfaction—then, modern psychology cannot find any justification for advising him to remain unhappy and nervous. But he should know that he has to take the chance of being socially handicapped; he cannot expect from other people a calm, philosophical, psycho-analytical view on this matter. He has to be ready to pay a price for his self-emancipation.

One thing, however, must be considered in all its consequences. A man or woman who is legally married, and has children, ought to know that very grave neuroses (mostly of the obsessional type) may be the destiny of children who have been brought up on the usual principles of sexual morality,[1] and who later realize that their parents have transgressed those principles. Dr. Stekel, during his life, had occasion several times to analyse parents, because of some minor neurosis, due to unfortunate marriage or sexual difficulties in their life; and later, children of the same parents, suffering from very grave obsessional neuroses, at times bordering even on schizophrenia, after such a discovery. Not in all cases, however, is such knowledge about the parents, however depressing to the child, followed by grave conditions. Some people may more or less overcome the shock. However, the possibility of a neurosis is by no means remote—and people should know this.

7. It is possible, for some individuals, to live a life of fair harmony and working efficiency without practical sexual life. It is possible for individuals whose sexual development—in its psychological aspect—has been suppressed during their childhood, or who from nature are endowed with but a weak urge, to carry their sexual suppression to the point of apparent entire absence of interest. This is true in spite of statements to the contrary on the part of many psycho-analysts. As a rule, they see patients who do suffer from mental conflicts, or from inefficient repressions; but their case-material hardly comprises people who are fairly well balanced and efficient in their daily life.

In many such cases there are present '*disguises of sexuality*'—certain habits, or fantasies, or activities which derive directly from the sexual instinct. But this is only the point of view of the psycho-analyst. In the general common-sense view of the layman there is no obvious trace of sexuality in such activities. And it would be a crime to destroy the harmony of such people—who are not less happy than the millions of their fellowmen who do live a normal sexual life—by deliberate scientific enlightenment about the disguised nature of their sexuality. It will be a great advance to relieve the minds of those who need such enlightenment, because they actually suffer, because they are in fact neurotic, and less efficient in life than they could be. But those others who are happy in their 'asexual' way, and amongst

[1] Cf. Ch. XXV (5), p. 142.

whom there are many deserving of public esteem because of their charitable, helpful, and socially pleasant behaviour, let them have their peace in their exceptional condition.

CHAPTER X

REGULATION AND REPRESSION OF TENDENCIES

1. THE operation of Instincts in man—let us here think first of the nutritional urge, leading to the supply of sufficient and proper food—comprises two antagonistically directed tendencies. The one is the positive urge, insisting on the satisfying of that biological necessity; and the other, complementary factor, results in restrictions and modifications of the very same urge and its satisfaction. This second factor has various sources and different aims. There are, first, considerations of healthy food, of enjoyable food, and of food to be taken at an appropriate time; this last factor means a time for meals, not interfering with other essential occupations, and also a period of comparative mental ease, enabling meals to be better enjoyed. The sources of another group of restrictions are external conditions, permitting and facilitating the satisfaction of the nutritional instinct. Certainly, the satisfaction of hunger should not lead to untoward consequences; it should comply with social habits, with the law and its regulations. The operation of this restrictive factor necessitates a part-repression of the first, urging, positive factor. The actual, satisfying behaviour of the individual is a resultant of the inter-activity of both trends.

The same simultaneousness of positive activity and repressive counter-activity obtains in the function of excretion. This complicate inter-activity of action and of regulative, adaptive inhibition is mostly realized by people only regarding the sphere of erotic, sexual tendencies. Yet, in fact, there is no function in man, whether physical or mental, whether mainly private or mainly social, which does not contain this bi-phasic [1] character. The repressive function is, in fact, immanent in every human manifestation of life.

There exists naturally a repression and neutralization of aggressive tendencies and of hatred. And there is frequently a very substantial repression of moral tendencies, of religious

[1] I.e. double-phased.

inclination, and in general, of the higher, so called 'anagogic' tendencies in man. Many a man represses his desire for going daily to church, and does so against his deepest liking, because his environment would not understand or appreciate it. And there are not a few people who, from one reason or another, would like to think of themselves as, and to pose as, apostolic and ascetic superhumans; but their common sense makes them conceal and combat this innermost wish and ideal of theirs.[1]

2. As is well known from psycho-analysis, the repressive function, whether it concerns the sexual or the aggressive tendencies, is not always efficient. The outcome of such inefficiency is the disposition to develop a neurosis when other difficulties of later life, conflicts, extraordinary burdens, etc., enter the stage of individual life. But I want to make it clear that this inefficiency of repression is as frequent with all the other human physiological and mental activities as it is with the two spheres mentioned. There certainly exists an inefficiency of the repression regulating evacuation; of the repression limiting and qualifying the individual's ambitions, his striving for prestige, his aiming at occupational and social results, and so on. The repressive function and its possible disturbances permeate the whole life. Counter-regulation and repression is as much a constant function of the human organization as is blood circulation, or alimentary assimilation, or hormonal stimulation; and as such it is subject to disturbances just as much as the other functions are.

It can be seen now how abundant are the possible sources for creating a neurotic disposition. The fields where repression operates, and where inefficiency of repression may occur, encompass, in fact, all the physiological motor and mental activities of man, both private and social. And if a man proves to be inefficient at carrying out his tasks in life and enjoying the gifts of his life, and at fitting himself into society; if a man proves to be neurotic (this expression means here any lack of adaptation), though the child, the predecessor of that particular man, seemed to be quite happy and promising—then let us think of all the possible fields of repression where this particular individual may have failed. And let us realize clearly how much help for the individual's particular functions can be given—or denied—by the environmental conditions in which he is expected to live, to develop and to carry on.

[1] Cf. Ch. XXI (6), p. 125.

No subsequent 'psycho-therapy' can entirely remove, for instance, nervous disturbances of the personality of the individual who, over a number of years, was never given the opportunity of taking his meals at ease and under external conditions appropriate to his taste and emotional requirements. And hardly any kind of psycho-therapy will be able substantially to help a neurotically developed individual who has been compelled, on innumerable occasions in the past, to miss going to a comfortable public lavatory. Or—to take a different sphere of life—if a sensitive child has to learn obedience through having to show respect to an unpleasant, neurotic teacher—and spends hours of his day in such an educational environment—no better circumstances later on can entirely repair the wrong committed against that child's developing personality. The necessary part-repression of his independence and resistance to education cannot in such a case be efficient. In brief, all our functions can be a source of non-efficient repression, if we extend this latter notion to the counter-regulating psycho-nervous processes in general. And I think the effect of such dysbalance between the operation of physiological functions and the complicated environmental considerations influencing that operation may also be a more or less significant source of a consequent neurotic make-up.

To summarize what has been explained in this chapter: There is practically no tendency and no function of man that is not greatly modified in its final manifestation by influences proceeding from the environment. The more or less smooth character of these processes constitutes an important buttress of the well-balanced personality; and similarly, disturbances of these processes may contribute to a neurotic character.

Repression should, therefore, be considered from this broader point of view. All those regulative counter-impulses which make the actions and physiological functions of the individual possible, expedient, and socially desirable, imply more or less repression of the original impulse, which aims at the unlimited fulfilment of that particular need, or at the carrying out of that particular action.

It goes without saying that neurotic traits which have their origin in such inefficient balance between functions and the related counter-regulations are hardly curable, or even capable of being understood, by means of the customary method and concepts of psycho-analysis. Prevention must be the chief task of medical science in these fields. But prevention here can only be effectuated by social and cultural reforms on a very broad scale, which permit a better spontaneity of the individual's life, both in its mental and in its physical aspects.

CHAPTER XI

THE SOCIAL PROCESS AND THE INDIVIDUAL

1. The individual is born with definite dispositions. This means that all that he is able to do in his later life is based on an inborn foundation. Yet the environment does much to educate him—i.e. to develop and to modify the natural raw material. The social environment—home, school, community—stimulates and facilitates the development of such qualities as, for instance, easy adaptability and tolerance ; it encourages the cultivation of skill and of personal independence ; it aims at the training of the individual in displaying, and cherishing, the sentiment of love ; it also requires of the individual that he should cultivate contempt for anti-social behaviour, whether within himself or in others. This educational process is commonly considered as natural and essential—and therefore as ' normal ' and easy.

The fact that many children are brought up by neurotic parents, markedly deficient in personal and educational qualities, and that their bodies and minds have to tolerate so many abnormal, undesirable influences, is not generally considered as a constant factor ; though in reality it is a very considerable one and its influence is very substantial. It is a self-blinding attitude on the part of any planned social organization, or any educational programme, not to take this constant disturbing factor into serious consideration.

In addition to all these things, and interwoven with them, comes the moulding influence of the wider social environment. For instance, if—as is the case today—everybody has to look after himself in the search for a satisfactory mode and standard of living, and if no Government is willing to procure or create a suitable job for him, then the educating parents and teacher will, more or less explicitly, but certainly implicitly, stress the importance of individual enterprise, of persistence in pursuing individual aims, and will praise more or less—but rather more than less—the efficiency of individuals who manage to achieve a good position and gain ample material means. The educating adults will enlarge on the success of those who manage to make thousands of small wage-earners work for them, whilst they themselves live in much greater personal freedom and with far wider scope for the gratification of their desires and needs of every sort.[1]

The particular structure of the economic and cultural organization exerts a substantial influence on the mind of the growing youth ; and this so-called *social process*, comprising all environmental influences, is part and parcel of those forces which shape the particular quality of the individual. If, for instance, the personal inclinations of a youth tend toward theoretical science, but, owing to the existence of his father's good business, he decides to grasp this latter opportunity, he will develop in himself any quality that is suitable for a good business man ; and he will, as a rule, repress most of that which could be useful for the career of a theoretician. In some cases there may be no apparent sign of an inefficient repression. But in other cases there ensues a peculiar personality-character ; the individual will prove quite good in working at his business, but yet he will appear somehow not well balanced, not quite pleasant, or not quite capable of spontaneity and happiness.

It is also obvious that the development of those character-traits which make the individual into a satisfactory, law-abiding citizen, is essentially part of the broader social process moulding the individual. And it is equally true that any Governmental system is able to modify the social process ; and also that the kind and amount and efficiency of individual repression of instincts can be, and are, essentially influenced by the particular ways of a communal organization and its administration. The following is what we mean.[2]

[1] Has not this been the predominant social outlook of most people in the United States for a long time now ? Its origin can be clearly seen in the lives the pioneers lived, the daily risks they were exposed to, and the boundless opportunities for personal advancement offered by a shifting frontier. Limitless opportunity, in this respect, was the firm foundation of the individualist economy of the United States. It explains, on the one hand, why, before the depression of 1929, trade unionism was regarded not just indifferently by the masses, but often with great hostility ; and on the other hand, it throws light on the popular feeling that an unemployed person had only himself to blame. The assumption in the former case was, and to a large degree still is, that any organization like a trade union, which causes men to agree to certain conditions of work, unnecessarily and wrongfully deprives people of that 'rugged individualism' which is the sacred and traditional index of the greatness of the United States ; and in the latter case, the inevitable assumption is that in a highly democratic country like the United States, abounding in opportunities, anybody who does not 'get on' must be highly deficient in 'guts' or common sense or the will to work. Such a person thus has only himself to blame. The absence of social security measures on a federal basis, until recently, illustrates this description, and well explains why the 'successful man' holds such a central position on the stage of American life.—*D.R.*

[2] Cf. Ch. XII.

2. A State-idea which is based on the sovereignty of the State (not the people), and on the absolute priority of State prestige, cannot but have a psychologically discouraging and burdening influence on the individual's personality ; and it has, in fact, manifested this influence. You will find how general has been the resentment at all times, and in various substantial strata of the population, against their particular Government, because the State as such, i.e. the Government of the day, is not interested in their ' private life ', and does not attempt everything possible to find suitable employment for each individual—and yet, with undue seriousness, condemns minor, formal offences, employing for this end the intelligence and the time of the Civil Servant.

The reader may be reminded of what has been explained in Chapter VI about the intensity of the task which the psyche of every child has to carry out in his adaptation of himself to the educational restrictions and to the authority of his parents. This process, and especially that part of it which is concerned with the task of successful repression of resentment of the parental authority and even of hatred of the parents, is carried over into the subconscious mental life of the adult. The mental personality of the adult thus needs a certain inner freedom for overcoming the infantile grudge against past educational hardships. But there is substantial pressure on men's minds from the existing social and Governmental system, and this pressure intensifies rather than relieves the effect of infantile psychic difficulties. When in later life the growing adolescent or the adult has first to face his state of unfreedom resulting from an unsatisfactory social system, when he realizes that he is the much weaker partner confronted by others who are financially and positionally stronger, then the ' digestion ' of his infantile father-complex may create more difficulties for his subconscious than it would if he felt that now, after having overcome the age of childish dependence, he was becoming a truly appreciated and at least mentally independent citizen of the State-family.

Naturally, there must also be a more or less substantial repression of resentment against the restrictions from social sources and against those originating in the particular—often only formal—regulations of the law. And the efficiency of this repression—which results in the social adaptation—is dependent on the anticipatory feeling with which the citizen-individual accepts his Government and its activities, on the feeling with which he accepts the particular State-organization and the particular State-ideology of his country. On the other hand, there is no doubt that a more harmonious attitude of the psyche in respect of intimate family problems and the intra-psychic [1] complexes connected with them, particularly with regard to the child-parent relations of the individual, must necessarily affect the ease or the difficulty of the broader social adaptation. This aspect has been recognized from the early stages of psycho-analytical research. And it has been generally assumed that the State-authority is, as it were, a branch-sphere or an extension of the parental authority ; and that the quality of the psychic attitude of the individual toward his parents and educators repeats itself, in different degrees, in his attitude toward the State-authority and toward society in general.

The present author thinks, however, that this simple conception calls for further remark in the light of various individual psycho-analyses. There is not infrequently a very ready acceptance of State-authority in people who consciously resent the authority of their parents. There are other people who become revolutionaries from a similar resentment. And finally, there are people whose attitude toward the State is indifferent, and only moulded by the actual necessities of an at least superficial adaptation, though they do suffer substantially from a difficulty of their parental relationship.

In the members of this third group it appears as if a social sense or deeper appreciation of a State-organization in general could not develop, owing to their neurotic condition in respect of their parental complex. The members of the first group react as if their attitude is : " Becasue my parents have hurt me, I prefer to be the obedient subordinate of any other master—the foreman, the head of the office, or the State in general." It is the attitude of a sensitive girl, deeply hurt and full of resentment and spite against her parents for their interference with her liberty, who decides to leave her comfortable home and become a housemaid or a nurse, submitting to the stricter discipline of such a position. It is easier, that is to say, for people of a certain type to bear the burden of restrictions imposed by those whom they do not love with the intensity and the irrational quality of infantile, elementary emotional tendencies. There is, perhaps, no necessity to enlarge on this point : these few remarks may suffice to make clear the mutual influence between the social process and the private mental spheres of the individual, and to indicate the variations of this interactivity.

It will be explained in Chapter XIII [2] that the necessary

[1] Cf. Ch. VI. [2] Cf. p. 78.

identification of the individual with his fellowmen can be accomplished with greater ease or greater difficulty according to the position that the individual has, or feels he has, within the existing social organization.

To summarize briefly : we have reason to assume that the particular social, cultural, and economic organization may influence the subconscious mental mechanism of the individual, by facilitating or hampering the solution of his most private and most delicate intra-physic emotional problems.

I have compared the analyses of five patients who were naturalized British citizens, and who in early childhood had emigrated from the same country. The parents of two patients were very successful from the very start ; whilst the parents of the other three had difficulties to overcome—more or less the same difficulties in each case. Owing to this fact, the home conditions of these three patients showed striking similarities. (For obvious reasons I am not in a position to go into the details.) Now, though these three men belonged to different personality-types, the specific colouring of their Oedipus-conflict, i.e. their specific reactions toward the authority of the father, appeared almost identical. And this was probably due to the similarity of certain environmental conditions—which, again, I cannot describe. The father-conflict of the two patients first mentioned assumed a quite different form, owing to the different social and economic standing of their parents.

3. What is called the experience of happiness is a highly subjective factor. It depends on the extent and depth of satisfaction of personal needs and individual aims. The elementary physiological needs and aims of various individuals are more or less uniform ; though, for instance, there may be marked differences in people's taste with regard to such things as the circumstances in which they take their meals. One person's psyche requires a more nicely laid table or tastier food, or a cosier or more decorative environment on the whole, than does the psyche of other persons, who wish more for lively company to add enjoyment to their meals. The particular circumstances of feeding may be of far greater significance for the individual's general behaviour than people think. The more or less satisfactory compliance with their individual requirements in this respect may make people more or less calm and contented for the rest of the day.

Far more subtle, however, are the individual differences as

to the general aims of life, as to the complex spheres of occupation, family and love-life, entertainment and rest. In many things the individual has to adapt himself to the possibilities, and to general customs and tastes ; and he is fully able to do so by virtue of the normal elasticity of his psyche. We can briefly state a provisional formula of happiness by saying that it is a product of two factors ; that which a person requires to satisfy his elementary and his more refined needs on the one hand, and, on the other, the amount and degree of what he has actually succeeded in obtaining, constitute two poles, the smallness of the gap between them being the measure of subjective satisfaction. But we have to go more exactly into the examination of this problem.

That which a person requires—mentally and physically—is not a static, not an absolutely rigid sum-total of things. The average individual's desirable aim in life is always such as to fit in, in a more or less advantageous way, with the social organization. To be or to have what brings appreciation from others, and to avoid possessing or being what would be followed by disfavour, contempt, and condemnation, is a very important viewpoint of the average individual in determining his aims in life. One may, for instance, in accordance with one's particular mental make-up, feel like living in solitude or amid simple conditions, but the realization of the extraordinary character of this subjective wish-pattern may be strong enough to effectuate the abandonment of such a primary aim in life. The same consideration applies, of course, to the value set upon financial power. The value is certainly determined by the actual economic significance of money and capital, and not primarily by elementary human nature.

The particular conditions in society, and the education of the individual, but not less the degree of normal independence of his mind, or, alternatively, the presence of an inferiority complex or of other neurotic traits in him, may substantially decide the manifested trends and aims of his wishing and striving. In the final outcome it is the dynamic power of these mental forces that decides his subjective satisfaction. The proportion above mentioned, between the things aimed at and those attained, is therefore not necessarily an index of the amount and depth of happiness of that individual. It is the psychic urgency of the particular wish that matters. One can share and display the conventional desire for much money ; but the fulfilment of it may not be absolutely necessary to satisfy one's mind and to overcome one's particular feeling of insecurity and inferiority. Deep down in his mind, a man may crave more substantially for quiet happiness in family life—and then, though there may be a gap between the financial goals aimed at and actually attained, the tension between the two poles may not be increased to a degree that would make him suffer.

One man's inferiority complex may be of such a kind that he wishes at all costs to have a nice-looking wife, admired by a great number of other people ; though she may not attain his standards —to which he attaches importance—of decency or average intelligence. Yet, the factor first mentioned may have a neurotically strong energetic charge in him ; and he may sacrifice everything else to satisfy this wish. Or, alternatively, if his common sense or his regard for family traditions forces him to consider the other factors—the defects of the wife of his desire—he may actually suffer from the ' gap ' owing to the ' polar tension '. I have chosen such an instance, since it may illustrate the interactivity of environmental, i.e. social influences, and individual, neurotic ones, together deciding the inner mental aim of an individual.

The above instance refers to a patient of mine. I happen to know something about the particular stages of his psycho-affective development. He was one of six children ; his mother frequently suffered from melancholic depressions ; the father appeared to be an irritable man, though kind-hearted. The children were brought up on very strict religious lines ; some of the brothers and sisters took things more easily, and developed into friendly, cheerful individuals. My patient, however, had apparently been of a quite different nature ; he took the strict principles of his religion very seriously, and spent much time reading theology and the philosophy of ethics. There was one very important impression in his life. He thought once, as a boy of eleven, that his mother, whilst travelling with him from their village to town, spoke too intimately to the driver ; perhaps even about her married life. This made the boy doubt the moral integrity of his mother—this was, however, only his own subjective interpretation—and subsequently he started *to doubt the absolute character of ethics altogether*. This idea became an obsession. He suffered much from religious conflicts, too ; he professed to be atheistic, and still could never feel satisfied about the philosophy of ethics.

He also always wanted to have a beautiful and healthy-looking wife—in order, I think, to counteract the recollection of his mother, who was of rather a ' common ' type, dull and ailing too. He frequently indulged in day-dreams, imagining how all the men in the town in which he was going to settle would admire him for his wife. This was apparently meant to overcome his own particularly strong feeling of inferiority. He then actually married a woman of very attractive appearance, but infinitely simple in outlook. He never admitted to himself that he, the man who used to buy heaps of philosophical books, could not be happy with such a life-partner. He went from analyst to analyst with his obsessional trouble ; but after a few conversations he usually discontinued the analysis. It was a fact, however, that, owing to his peculiarities and his serious manner, his friends and his employers preferred his wife as company, and readily forgave her superficial, simple structure of mind. This I knew from the psycho-analysis of a fellow-worker of his. Thus his choice of a wife who was beautiful and healthy, though unintelligent, proved to be advantageous to him from the social point of view ; but his choice was also markedly influenced by the deeper tendency to overcome the recollection of his simple-looking and sick mother.

The above instance is naturally a psycho-pathological one. But the inter-activity of forces, deciding the steps of the individual, is aptly illustrated. Had this man lived in a society in which it was the intellectual level of a person, and his working capacity, that mattered chiefly, he would have had more self-confidence, since he was an able worker in his occupation. He would have been able to rely more on his own qualities than on the beauty of his future wife ; and he might have been able to overcome that particular desire of ' painting out ' the recollection of his mother. Or he would probably have given to his mother-conflict a different expression—striving for an exceptionally clever wife, even if not so attractive in appearance as to be admired by strange men. All this is naturally only interpretation and a conclusion of the analyst. And any interpretation may be either approximately right or, perhaps even more frequently, essentially mistaken. However, the deeper understanding of what psycho-analysis and its related sciences state about the significance of infantile traumas, and about the undue increase from environmental sources of a child's natural inferiority feelings, the proper understanding and more modern interpretation[1] of these findings, together with the study of the history of civilization, certainly suggests the conclusion that particular environmental and social influences may deeply

[1] That is, advancing beyond the classical psycho-analytical explanations of the Freudian school.

affect the individual's make-up, the qualities of his ambitions, and the ways in which he tries to realize them and to overcome his fears and his feelings of insecurity, and to attain the desirable means within his reach of securing social success and private happiness.

4. The feeling of insecurity, of an unsatisfactory position within the family and society, and a sense of inferiority of intellectual capacity—these things create in many young individuals an insatiable desire for sexual experiences. The reverse phenomenon also occurs. The pressure of social difficulties and the resultant feeling of personal inferiority depress, in many sensitive, introvert types, the desirable development of their love-faculty. Yet in the extravert type, in young individuals with a healthy life-instinct, deficiencies in education, and a family environment without stability and peace, may be followed by an urge toward numerous ephemeral love-relationships. Their psyche craves for something deeper, which, however, they cannot easily attain. Their parents live in poverty and unrest ; their own social future is not well prepared by education of their mind and heart ; they see everywhere the threat of frustration, and difficulty in competing with influential and better-educated fellow-beings. To wait until sustained effort could secure them a fairly satisfactory position, economic and social, and enable them to enter into a marriage that holds out the promise of an average peace and standard of life—such waiting and hoping requires some energy, endurance, firmness of character, and natural intelligence. Obviously the number of those in possession of such qualities is not larger than the number of those who are lacking in them and who submit easily to the temptations of the immediate present. Improved social conditions could certainly change the destiny of many individuals who, when growing older and more mature, greatly deplore the thoughtless course started in earlier life.

In many cases it is not so much the actual parental control of the adolescent youth that prevents an early entanglement in undesirable types of sex-relationship. It is largely the emotional satisfaction from the family atmosphere that contributes to the balance of the emotion-ego of the youth. The sexual feeling and the general emotional function lie on the same keyboard of the psyche ; and in many individuals a disharmony in general emotionality is followed by a disharmonic emergence of sex. It is, however, not the task of the family environment to inhibit the development of libidinal feeling and interest, either by moralistic strictness or by increasing the ties of family fixation. The desirable type of family life gives automatic protection against an easy yielding to the opportunities of ill-considered love-relationships.

It is now easier to see where the question of social reform comes in. The inner structure of the family, provided that there is not much of inherited psychopathic elements in the members, depends largely on general financial and cultural conditions, as well as on the quality of the knowledge and views that guide the average human being in living and in his outlook on life.

This is not simply theoretical discussion and abstract generalization. In individual cases of young neurotics or delinquents a transfer into a quite different family circle, and the imparting of healthy views to the patient in question, has succeeded in diverting the personality in desirable directions. I do not want to raise excessive hopes in the case of all unbridled young people with excessive innate psychopathic inclinations, even if ' analysed ' and then placed in a different environment, cultural and economic. But the number of border-line cases, in which the inborn disposition toward undesirable behaviour is still largely dependent on an intensifying environmental factor in order to become manifest and considerable, is large enough to merit the attention of the social reformer. And amongst these types with a slight ' criminal disposition ' are many kind-hearted and even talented individuals, whom it is a pity to lose for the benefit of society and for their own satisfactory life.

5. There is one more very important point to discuss about the elementary conditions of happiness, in so far as it is affected by the social process—the factor of the inborn constitution of the individual. No doubt the nervous systems of different people, and the quality of the continuous processes of stimulation, of the impulses and counter-impulses, occurring within the nervous cells and within the intangible ' Mind ', vary greatly. There are psycho-somatic constitutions in which there is, from birth, always some disharmony, more or less ' nervous and mental indigestion ' ; such a person never feels quite at ease, because his ' nervous metabolism ' works under strain, owing to constitutional weakness. This fact, naturally, also increases his difficulties in social adaptation, in smoothly overcoming disappointments, and in repressing resentment and hatred ; and it acts as an impediment to the growth in him of the necessary minimum of optimism.

Such a person might feel more at home, and might develop better, in a social system in which everybody can be sure of his due place without belonging to a privileged class, or possessing aggressiveness enough to secure a ' good seat ' in the theatre of life. In such a society his constitutional nervous weakness would have no particular significance for such a person—there would be no necessity for him to develop those different compensatory neurotic or asocial trends, described so aptly by Adler. An individual can become unsocial, suspicious, excessively thrifty, simply because his psyche is trying to over-compensate his inner feeling of insecurity. Solitude saves the weak individual from much disappointment, and from attacks on his pride. Suspicion is similarly meant to forestall social defeats. The hoarding of money may give the feeling of more or less power ; and the reluctance to spend it may be essentially a symbolic attitude of not ' giving oneself ', of remaining detached from the crowd of fellow-beings, and their needs, and thus protected from their calls upon one.

It is worth while to take seriously these psychological assumptions, and to venture on a thoroughgoing social reform, in the hope of attaining more happiness for the next generation. Man will never change his essential nature, but in his reactions he can certainly change. The term ' reactions ' implies a feeling experienced, and a behaviour displayed, in response to environmental occurrences. Whatever the individual does from subjective and selfish motives, he has more or less to modify and to colour his particular way of acting, and even of feeling and thinking, according to environmental conditions. And these acts of his, carried out under this influence of environmental factors on his psyche, we call ' reactions ' ; and it is also assumed that this particular aspect of the personality is and can be, to a substantial degree, modified, and therefore could be modified in a more or less planned manner.

I do not wish to overstress the possibilities of such ' planned rearing ' of individuals into desirable personality-types. I still think that inborn dispositions (so-called instincts) of eternal validity are the basis, and the limiting factors, of the human personality. What *has*, however, changed in man during history is the consequence of his increased knowledge of Nature and of his developed individuality. The social setting of the human species has certainly undergone a marked development ; and accordingly we may assume that that part of human behaviour which is closely related to the environment is capable of adaptation. The present author, however, is inclined to think that that social structure, that particular reform in social life, is the more advanced one, which is the more accomplished in helping the individual to live in accordance with his inborn dispositions, to satisfy them and *to develop them.* There is only one additional remark to be made : The potential dispositions of man are far richer than is assumed by the too simplified conceptions on human instincts. For instance, morality, refined love, and the social sense,[1] are also part of the ' instinctual ' dispositions in man. And the social backwardness of past centuries was mainly manifested by the utter disregard for the individual and his differentiated dispositions.[2] The author is aware that this conception of his may evoke the opposition of many modern authors.

6. People reading the current psycho-analytical explanations of social phenomena frequently gain a somewhat unpleasant impression from them—that of an attempt to reduce all that is high and valuable for morality and social adaptation to repressed ' wrong instinctual tendencies ' of man. They are not entirely mistaken with regard to the true opinion of several authors. But they are certainly mistaken with regard to other not less up-to-date psychologists. I may refer, for instance, to what has been suggested above—that all that is refined in man is also part and parcel of his innate and ancient potential disposition.[3] The contribution of repressions, and of transformations of instinctual or reactive attitudes into socially and ethically approved behaviour, does not mean more than a refinement of certain biological energies and dispositions and their utilization in other fields and for other aims. What happens in these so-called sublimating spheres is absolutely comparable with that eternal process carried out by Nature, the utilizing of waste products of animate and inanimate life for the renewed growth of rich and beautiful natural produces. It is also comparable to that modern process of planned economy in which every sort of scrap is considered as a source of future new production; as a source which is not merely incidental, but relied upon from the very start as an essential element of the continual process of regeneration subsidiary to production.

[1] The postulate of social justice is very old in history of mankind.

[2] This expression denotes the complicated ' many-sidedness ' of human tendencies, capable of various specialized modifications.

[3] Some authors express their belief that acquired, i.e. non-ancient, dispositions too can be transmitted in the course of generations. See *Habit and Heritage*, by Fred. Wood Jones, 1943.

CHAPTER XII

THE GOVERNMENT AND THE CITIZEN

1. THE State-organization, even the most up-to-date, is essentially concerned with the ' citizen ', but hardly in general with the human ' individual '. Its legislation and regulations aim at the maintenance of public order. Agriculture, industrial production, craftsmanship and business, though carried on by private citizens and primarily from private motives, fall within the scope of the interest of the State, since the exchange and smooth distribution of different goods among the population are elementary necessities of a regulated public life.

There is also a certain control of traffic and travel, of housing and of public hygiene. And there is a due emphasis on the spheres of education and art, providing under present conditions for the higher intellectual and emotional requirements of the population. A system of laws regulates certain, though limited, aspects of inter-personal life, of local administration, and of the institution of marriage. But with the innermost private happiness or unhappiness of the individual and of the family, the State is not concerned. The individual is allowed to shape his course in life and to strive and struggle for his livelihood—that is, to look after his own physical and mental satisfaction. The system of laws regulates, to a certain extent, the simultaneous life-process of the various individual members of the population, in competition with one another. Murder, robbery, fraudulence, and public scandals, and to a small degree even attacks on the personal honour of the individual, are guarded against by the deterrent of subsequent legal retribution.

The State says in effect : " You may take from life all you want, and especially as much as you can by your individual skill, so long as you keep my regulations, so long as you do not transgress the letter of the law." But whether the spirit of the law is maintained or not, has not so far seriously concerned the State. The wise comments of indignant judges at court proceedings and the occasional solemn pronouncements of individual members of the Government, the Churches, and the Universities, are, I think, not sufficient proofs of the State's fundamental interest in and active concern with the human or inhuman spirit of public life ; they do not reveal sufficiently serious State concern with the promotion of individual happiness and the prevention of avoidable individual suffering in mind and body.

One can be happy or unhappy ; one can suffer from endless mental conflicts ; one can be exposed to continuous attacks on one's aims, continual challenges to one's goodwill and optimism. One can succeed or fail in one's relationship with relatives or friends. One can commit endless mistakes from emotional weakness or from intellectual ignorance, and bear—for oneself alone—the natural consequences of any unguarded step. One is entitled to do all this ; one is permitted to endure years, even a lifetime, of continuous dysbalance, sorrow and regret. The State does not compel its officials to care for a man's private condition.

There is the greatest possible 'democratic' freedom in this respect. Yet, surely, in keeping with the many and great advances in science, both social and general, many things could be prevented or remedied by the State, which the individual has neither the means nor the executive power to avoid or to put right. Many hours of useless worry on his part could then be devoted instead to useful or enjoyable activity.

The provision for education, public assistance, public comfort, for the enjoyment of the higher or more primitive arts, for public baths and public parks and so on, is simply a 'departmental activity' of the State.[1] But the basic idea of the State-organization is not the individual's happiness, not his physical and mental well-being, but essentially the prestige, or at least the authority, of the State [2] and a regulated, prosperous national life in general,

[1] Even if the actual administration of a State *was* mainly devoted to general social welfare and only a small part of it to the traditional political and international institutions, the basic State-idea would still not be 'the greatest happiness of the the greatest number'. So long, for instance, as it is legal for a Government to take even *one* decision expressive mainly of the traditional State prestige, a decision which may be economically or emotionally beneficial to 'leading circles' but which pays no thought to the interest of the broad masses ; so long as it is legal to utilize public means, the means of the country as a whole, for purposes which have no bearing at all on the above ideal of 'just distribution'—the sociological writer is justified in advocating a reformed State-idea. Naturally the Utopian character of such suggestions, so far as the immediate future is concerned, and of the perfect materialization of such a State-administration at any period of human history, is as clear to the author as to his critics. But he hopes to find general assent to the view that desirable principles, if once clearly recognized, ought to be presented always in their maximal purity. This makes possible a true measure of existing conditions. There must also be a continual incentive to further improvements, and to a periodical overhaul of conditions. Similarly, when we speak about justice or morality, we envisage these concepts in their absolute purity, in order to have a measure, and at the same time an ideal, for the actual life, so abounding in deficiencies.—S. L.

[2] The basic idea of a State-organization naturally depends on the particular State in question, its economic structure, its geographical position, and its historical tradition. Some States, in virtue of the foregoing reasons, stress the prestige of the State much more than others. The same is true of the insistence on the authority of the State. But I think there is, and has been, a qualitative difference in the place of State prestige in Germany and Japan, as compared to Great Britain. The Englishman very rarely approaches the name and idea of the State 'on his knees'. One of the things that most surprise foreigners about Great Britain is the indifference, often the humorous indifference, which the Englishman shows for the Royal Family and

which gives or denies the things needed by the individual according to its particular legal system as interpreted by the executive Civil Service.[1] The fundamental priority of the right of the mass of individuals to live happily, and to have the help of the whole State organization for that end, is a conception still largely alien to the present State-idea.

Why should it be impossible, for instance, to have a ministerial department earnestly concerned about the inner life of families ? Why should it be fantastic to imagine a Departmental Welfare Director who reviews reports showing how many working hours in this or that vital factory were lost in recent weeks owing to nervous breakdowns of girls, following their unsatisfactory home life, and who even thinks earnestly of possible improvements?

Parenthetically speaking : We psycho-analysts have known for a long time, and now it is being realized by general medicine, that a great number of individuals catch a cold, or even develop tonsilitis,[2] immediately after having experienced some extraordinary mental strain or conflict. It appears as if the resistive capacity of the body—so greatly dependent on the tone of the autonomic nervous system—may give way under such attacks on mental harmony. There is, however, another mental factor fairly well established in frequent cases. There is in man a tendency of self-destruction—its maximal manifestation is suicide —which may come into operation on occasions when life seems to offer insurmountable difficulties, or when it seems to a sensitive person that ' life is scarcely worth living '. The physical consequences may be a decrease of resistance against colds and infections.

I knew during my practice two outstanding instances of people who, in consequence of their unsolved ' complexes ', reacted every winter regularly with bronchitis of exceptional duration. One of these was a Civil Servant in a high position, who for years used to be absent from his work for weeks and months, and who regularly got run down whenever the idea of marriage cropped up. After analysis, and after abandoning all thought of marriage,

the Houses of Parliament, even in public, in striking contrast to the solemn attitude which the German traditionally adopts, in company, to the Fatherland. It is true that in the international sphere State prestige has been very important in all countries owing to the assumptions of international society, where military power and diplomatic prestige play such an important part.—D. R.

The author is concerned with State authority and State prestige only in so far as these factors may promote or restrict the well-being of the mass of ordinary citizens.—S. L.

[1] Cf. Ch. XXVI.

[2] Von Weitzsäcker recorded nearly 200 cases of tonsilitis developed after mental shocks or difficulties.

his yearly colds became just of average kind. Think of the social aspect of such occurrences. The other case was that of a scientist whose psycho-analysis, originally carried out because of impotency, led to his deliverance also from severe colds, which used to keep him really ill in bed for weeks, and away from his occupational obligations.

It is not necessary that such instances should be tackled only when the individual suffers from a breakdown, and has the good fortune to be advised on appropriate treatment—assuming that he also has the money and time for such treatment, entailing five analytical hours a week for about six months.

There is no way of coping satisfactorily with this problem other than to prevent, as far as possible, the development of deeper-going neuroses. This prevention is possible along the lines suggested in several parts of this volume. We have frankly to inform the public, and all the authorities dealing with the public medical service, that there is no financial possibility of providing psycho-therapeutic treatment of a sufficient degree for the general mass of neurotics, if we are called upon to deal with such serious and long-standing conditions as we do, as a rule, in our present practice. Apart from the great amount of time and effort necessary for such cases—and even for those considered as not complicated—and even if every therapist were in possession of the skilled technique of shortened analyses as advocated, for instance, by Stekel, there is another point which would present a substantial handicap in psycho-therapy carried out on behalf of a panel or the State panel system. If the financial contribution of the patient is not so great as to make him feel it a burden, one important aid to overcoming the so-called subconscious resistance against treatment will be missing ; the difficulties for treatment under such conditions are well known to every expert. It is, therefore, absolutely necessary that serious attention shall be paid to these suggestions aiming at early attention to people's conflicts and minor breakdowns.[1] This is not only a humanitarian gesture of the psychologist, but a serious problem facing the communal organization, in which people have not superfluous means, and at the same time need to work as regularly as possible.

2. The individual does not like to work for others. This is an elementary fact, a *primitive reaction*. It is the ' citizen ' who works

[1] At such an early stage the inner subconscious resistance against treatment is, in most cases, not yet firmly established ; and the question of expense may not come in such force on to the ' battle-field '.

and does his duty. As soon as the individual has to suffer intra-psychic difficulties he is often unable to summon up sufficient energy to persuade himself that he is ready to be a 'citizen'. And his 'social layer' is the first to break down. If, however, man could have a little more of individual love for being a citizen, we could safely assume that his work would less easily become tiresome to him, and his being a dutiful citizen, in whatever occupation, would be a more solid factor, supporting, propping up his personality, in spite of acute volcanic disturbances in its strictly private layers. We know, in fact, a few individuals to whom work, 'their work', meant so much that it could help them to tide over stormy moments in their intra-psychic life. But in the overwhelming majority of cases men do not feel so much at one with their occupation, since they feel their position in society, and, consequently, their work-contribution to society, as irksome and only enforced.

It is a very apt observation, made most clearly by a recent writer, Fromm,[1] that individual freedom of the kind prevailing in our democratic and capitalistic State-organization implicitly entails a certain mental isolation of the individual. He can do what he wants, but the others, too, do only what *they* want. We must agree that the State, as such, is far from being the 'family circle' for the individual.[2] But it could be different.

[1] *Fear of Freedom.*

[2] The divorce between the theory and the practice of a State-organization is usually, and always has been, very real; and people do not seem to realize the reason for it. It is one thing to preach pious principles which should be the basis of State practice, and quite another thing to translate such moral and verbal enthusiasms into the legal and administrative stuff from which decisions are drawn. If the week-end speeches of politicians in their constituencies were taken at the face-value of their idealistic content, the world of problems and unhappiness would be found to be fast disappearing. The difference between State theory and practice can be clearly seen in the United States. Anyone who contrasts the moral fervour, and the militant claims for 'individual liberty and human equality', of the Declaration of Independence and the Constitution, with the gross inequalities of American life, political and economic, and the absence of Federal and State means for ensuring individual security and family happiness, can see this plainly. The tradition of 'rugged individualism' of American society largely accounts for this.

I think, though, that it is an implicit assumption of more politicians and many more citizens in England than in the U.S.A. that the State should, and does as far as it can, try to ensure the 'greatest happiness of the greatest number'. The Beveridge Plan is one indication of this temper. This is all the more surprising since there is no written Constitution or recent document in English history that proclaims the importance of individual happiness and human equality; though what a politician thinks is conducive to community happiness, depends largely on where he comes from, what he does for a living, and the kind of economic society he lives in.

In the U.S.S.R. there appears to be a much more comprehensive attempt to see to "the fundamental priority of the right of the multitude of individuals to live happily and to have the help of the whole State organization for that end". Note this tendency in phrases like 'State Planning Commission', 'Planned Production for Community Consumption', and the important 'health and happiness' functions of the trade unions in the factories.—D. R.

The Catholic Church, for instance, and similarly every organized religious community, certainly gives more of this kind of support to the individual. It is true that it also asks for subordination and sacrifice, and places considerable restrictions on the freedom of movement of the members. Anti-religious sentiment, atheistic tendencies, crop up at certain moments in many believers' minds. And yet, undeniably, the individual is comforted by the knowledge of belonging to his religious body. The Church in general tries to be, and is to a greater extent than the State, the family of the individual.

We do not overlook the differences ; we do not overlook that statements and promises which are made by religion refer to metaphysical spheres, to God and heaven, and concern the immortal soul, and that, therefore, the mere assurance fills the mind with the happiness of the belief in and the enjoyment in advance of a condition which is bound to be concrete experience for the individual, once he becomes himself a spirit, rid of the burdens of its material frame. Whilst human expectations on earth demand immediate and tangible fulfilment, yet there is in fact far more pain and disappointment during life than satisfaction and fulfilment. But, all the same, the earthly administrators of religion definitely carry out their calling better than the mundane Governments, with their particular administrative procedures ; they show more personal interest and more equality of their interest in the various members of their particular denomination than is the case in the relationship of Government and citizen.

Most of what our modern State does for the citizen bears more the mark of charity or voluntary presents than that of natural shares. The idea of the State for the present-day man is not a 'cosy' one. In fact, many a citizen feels not quite 'at home' in his country. He may like his town, his fellow-citizens, and certain customs peculiar to his country. He will certainly like the existence of those legal and social institutions which enable him to earn, in a sufficient degree, his living, and which enable him to have his luxuries and pleasures. But I hardly believe that the number of citizens loving their Government and Governmental system is substantial. No wonder! The spiritual background of the State-idea so far hardly deserves such a sentiment of love ; it has not been capable of evoking, in the hearts of millions, such affection.

The humble and weak citizens, therefore, wish to say to their Governments : "Give us sufficient and suitable opportunity to work as long as we are physically fit; and let us live in humane conditions if we are incapable of working any more. Take away our hourly anxieties concerning the health, the occupational training, and the general human future of our children. You State! You have such means at your disposal to that end. Fight against unjustified prejudices; eliminate, as far as possible, conditions which lead to too much hypocrisy. Do not force, by social conditions and conventions, immature individuals into an early, unconsidered marriage, and do not force unfortunate young people to give birth to children who should never have started their 'unhappy walk' in the world. Free us from bureaucracy, from the general impersonal attitude of the administration. Give us science, information, enlightenment on every necessary matter of life. . . . In short, decrease the amount of our intra-psychic struggle; and utilize the energies so saved for common work, for general happiness, and for imposing the strong pressure of the law and public opinion on the individual, moulding him into a more tolerant and more kind, less neurotically selfish and less neurotically cruel being. For such a State-organization we should have true love."

CHAPTER XIII

THE SOCIAL FACULTY OF MAN

1. *Loneliness is the hunger of the 'social instinct'.* From time immemorial man has felt the necessity of living amongst, and with, fellow-beings. He needs them to supplement his own personality, i.e. to buttress up his own subjective and objective insufficiency; he needs them to enjoy his similarity to his fellowmen, and at the same time his awareness of difference from them. He requires his environment for satisfying his tendency for leading and ruling, and at the same time for satisfying that other, no less human, tendency of being led and ruled. And he needs his fellow-beings in order to irradiate them with his appreciation and love; and to receive from them the same sentimental gifts for his own psyche.

The urge of this social instinct is unceasing. This can be seen, for instance, in children. They may quarrel and hurt each other, and feel hurt—and yet at the next moment they are together again, laughing, playing, or teasing and attacking each other. And similar phenomena may be observed in simple people, who have not acquired much of that studied pride and self-esteem which compels most of us to harbour and cultivate resentment against those who have hurt us, or have shown manifest insincerity or selfishness. These less sophisticated people vehemently display their dissatisfaction and aggressive attitude toward those who annoy them ; but soon, without much embarrassment, they approach each other again as if nothing had happened. They may at times deceive themselves as to the true motives of their readiness to forgive. They may make themselves believe that practical interests, and even selfishness, account for their undignified behaviour, and that it is only from such 'ulterior' motives that they feign friendship toward their 'adversaries' who happen to be their neighbours. But we feel certain that at the back of their studied self-interpretation there is the elementary urge of their *social sense*, driving them toward forgiveness and active manifestation of friendliness.

2. It is not only an incidental occurrence in the world of man that some people prove stronger, imposing their will and guidance and their personal interests on others ; whilst those who are weaker have to give in. The primitive layers of the psyche are endowed by nature with an appropriate tendency toward giving in, toward accepting domination or suppression. The psychic apparatus is thus fitted to meet these inescapable facts of life. This elementary tendency in man is genuinely satisfied when he is being ruled and suppressed ; since there is, in fact, a kind of innate instinct in him toward submission too. The masochist, who derives even erotic pleasure from the cruel or even torturing behaviour of his counterpart the sadist, is essentially not an exceptional figure. Almost everybody is capable of deriving a specific satisfaction from submission ; provided that he meets the one supreme personality who is capable of evoking in him (and it may well be in him only) this acceptance of rule, and even of painful exploitation. True, in many so-called normals the sense of self-assertion and self-esteem has first to be broken down and eliminated, in order to free the way for the emergence of this other characteristic, the primitive masochism.[1] But in the spheres of love proper there are not infrequently similar manifestations observable. Many a man, originally sure of his emotional independence and keen on being himself first approached and appreciated by a

[1] This denotes the emotional satisfaction by submission of the deep layers of the mind, but with the exclusion of any manifest sexual tinge, such as exists in the case of the masochist proper.

member of the other sex, at some time suddenly finds himself deeply devoted to a woman who seems specifically fitted to call into play this faculty of submissive devotion, pushing into the background the previous, not less genuine, independence of spirit. And the same occurs with some women. Naturally this phenomenon is not quite the same as the above tendency of servile submission ; one understands better a devotion displayed in a condition of deep and satisfying love-relation. However, the essential difference between the two instances, I think, is the fact that we are better able to understand the one possibility, and are reluctant to acknowledge the existence of the other, less dignified one. Satisfaction of a submissive tendency does not necessarily imply 'to be happy and satisfied'. What is meant is the satisfaction of a part-tendency of the deeper psyche. Owing to this satisfaction, which is more than a mere 'putting up with' something, the personality is not bound to suffer a total breakdown in the case of a continuous suppression. This evil consequence would have to ensue if the oppressed individual could only 'put up with' his condition, only spend energy on tolerating it, without being compensated by some sort of intra-psychic satisfaction.

No doubt the history of the last two decades has sufficiently illustrated the existence of this almost loving submission by young men to a brutal leader. It is possible to distinguish, during careful analysis, this submissive tendency and the satisfaction derived from it on the one hand, and that attitude of devotion which is derived from veiled and modified homosexual tendencies in connexion with the brutal and admired leader. True, in the spheres of overt manifestation the emotions from both sources work closely tied up to one sentiment.

Pathological phenomena in mental life are only distortions and one-sided accentuations of normal tendencies. And the purpose of the above excursions has been simply to illustrate better the genuine principal item of the discussion in this chapter. The social sense, as has been said, is such an elementary factor in present-day man's make-up, that society could certainly make use of it in a far more intensive, more beneficial, and more dignified manner.

3. There are human qualities and faculties which, though constant components of the personality, appear to be operative only when an appropriate situation evokes them or requires their manifestation. A great deal of human activity, mental and physical,

occurs in response to environmental conditions. Human skill and invention, the infinite wealth of ideas, and the great variety of modes of behaviour, are only to a small part stimulated primarily by inner needs ; mostly they are manifested in response to environmental conditions, both physical and social. From this angle the greatest part of individual psychology is in fact social psychology.

The manifestations of mass psychology merit special attention. There are modes of behaviour which the individual displays only when he is a member of a mass ; when he is no longer an individual member of a community, but merely a standardized unit of a mass, living under the influence of a mass-emotion. Every individual has in himself the potential disposition to become such a mass-atom, and to display an appropriate behaviour. But until this particular feeling and behaving does take place, the individual is, as a rule, quite unaware of bearing in himself this potential mass-psyche. The occasion has first to come, the creation of the mass has to take place ; and the emergence and development of the mass-psyche in the individual follows immediately.

Though not only deplorable manifestations of destruction and cruelty, but much progress in human history, has occurred through the powerful medium of the mass-psyche, through mass-enthusiasm, the mass-formation always clearly betrays its derivation from primitive, prehistoric stages of human history. There is always something irrational, chiefly emotional, in mass-manifestations ; and there is also an easy response to the suggestions of a leader, because the critical faculty and awareness of individuality in the members of the mass has receded into the background.

The satisfaction from submission, from largely surrendering one's individuality—this phenomenon, dealt with above, is clearly operative in the mass-formation. There is no need to think necessarily of a fanatical leader, inspiring and inciting a mass. The enthusiasm manifested at a musical concert, a theatrical performance, a religious or political meeting, contains similarly this factor of submission. Only here it is an idea, a principle, a cultural element, that is not only enjoyed and approved by the mass, but is at the same time an overpowering factor during the period of the mass-creation.

It seems as if the readiness to form masses is directly proportionate to the amount of instinctual repression in the individuals. Organized religious ideologies, for instance, powerfully repress the instincts of sex and aggression. And this instinctual repression results, to a certain degree, in a ' suppression ' of the personality, making the person less individual and more a type-unit. *It is the resulting suppression of the individual that, in the opinion of the author, makes for ready and intense mass-manifestation.* Freud [1] had clearly seen that there is a kind of 'libidinal tie' between the members of a group. But certainly there is much more than elementary libido at the base of mass-formation in the sense dealt with here. The enthusiasm, or the wildness, of masses—i.e. of short-lived emotional groups—is based on a transformation of the factor of individuality; it is directly proportional to the suppression of individuity.[2] Instinctual suppression and repression has only a bearing on the mass-psyche of the individual in so far as his actual individuity is affected by it. An instinctual suppression, which does not interfere too much with the individuity, does not increase the average susceptibility of the individual for mass-emotion, whether base or lofty.

This is the point at which a mass-formation of civilized social strata resembles the mass-manifestations of 'sub-cultural' primitive groups. The members of groups of a lower culture are certainly less restricted in the spheres of manifested sex and aggression; or, more correctly, they are not restricted in the same ways as the members of a civilized stratum. But the suppression of the individual personality is very substantial in savage or sub-cultural societies (and under a dictatorship too). The emotional ego of their members is not well developed; it is dynamically in much the same unfavourable condition as if subjected to instinctual suppression and as if suffering from unsuccessful repression of the type found in our current cultural pattern.

The significance of mass-situations for the life of a society is naturally great. And the problem consists in exploring the conditions which are bound to increase idealistic and creative mass-manifestations and decrease the tendency to the formation of 'wild masses'. It appears that the suppression of the individual's personality, to a degree optimal for the communal interest, still leaves enough integrity of the personality to maintain the necessary self-esteem and also the due appreciation of the fellow-being living in the same circumstances. Two slaves can pity each other and enter into a plot against their oppressor. But their psyche will never carry out the normal identification with each other. There is little in the personality of the one slave with which his fellow-sufferer will wish to identify himself. In

[1] *Group Psychology*, 1921. (English translation by James Strachey, 1940.)
[2] Individuity=the particular personality of the individual.

true identification there is an attempt at enrichment of one's own mental structure through incorporating into oneself the image of the fellow-personality.[1] But under conditions of 'optimal suppression of individuality' the retained degree of self-esteem enables the individual to appreciate the personality of his fellow-beings, to identify himself with them, and to be ready for 'enthusiastic mass-formation', but hardly for the creation of 'unbridled masses' charged with the spirit of destruction.[2]

4. In the course of communal life there is a mutual identification of the members of society ; and this emotional tie is one of the chief factors that make collaboration and mutual consideration possible. The external pressure of the law, and the recognition of social necessities in general, are responded to on the part of the individual by the operation of this intra-psychic process of identification ; and this process is followed by the acceptance by the individual of subjection to the claims, in return for the benefits, of the communal organization—together with his fellow-citizens, with whom he identifies himself.

Now, it is easy to see that this process of identification must necessarily operate better when there exists, within the community, a certain genuine equality in the social and legal position of the members ; i.e. when the individual feels that in social significance, in rights and burdens, in the possibilities of inner spontaneity and happiness, there are no very marked differences, no such differences as are caused by unjust distribution of possibilities and means. And, conversely, there must be a great deal of inner resistance against this desirable process of identification if the individual knows that the opposite is the case ; and especially if he also feels that unrestricted competition and complete freedom of individual enterprise automatically makes one individual the potential enemy of the other. This latter factor is naturally inevitable in our society. But it is well to be aware of it, and to attempt to compensate the individual for its existence by other social improvements ; thus showing unequivocally to the citizen that the State regrets, as it were, any inconvenience or suffering ensuing from the defective character of the existing social organization. Let us recall the far more provident—and

[1] See Ch. VI (4).

[2] Just as repression can be unsuccessful, so some identifications in fact facilitate neurotic dysbalance. But the two processes are primarily instruments of mental regulation and of growth respectively.

surely more efficient—attitude of the Church in past centuries, in keeping down so much individualism and envy by assuring all her members of her equally deep love and care for the immortal soul of each one of them. In this belief, in past centuries, the poorest peasant or serf could meet his lord and tyrant at the Sunday service with his mind at rest, and could even feel more or less true devotion for him. The community of their religious spheres and of metaphysical hopes straightened out much of their differences.

5. There are difficult [1] 'social characters'.[2] There are people, that is to say, who are unable to feel and to behave as if in genuine need of fellow-beings. There are people to whom everybody outside their intimate family circle is a 'stranger' accepted only 'on sufferance'. There are individuals who, when analysed, are sincere enough to declare that they have no belief in altruism, in 'love for others', and who doubt the existence of any true satisfaction in doing what is kind and helpful to others. In this respect much, very much, depends on the years of earliest development in the life of the child. Lack of true love and understanding, terror in education, cold suppression of the child's natural inclination to the early manifestations of infantile sexuality, and yet other factors not easily described to the non-expert, may exert a substantially distorting influence on the development of the social character. In this sense, difficulties of social, inter-human relations are just as much 'neuroses' for the psychiatrist as are anxiety-states, sexual neuroses, obsessions, etc. The practical difference lies in the fact that neuroses of the social sense are almost impossible to eliminate in later life. The first prerequisite of a successful psychological treatment is that the patient suffers from his neurosis. But such individuals rarely suffer enough from their 'queer' or anti-social nature to be ready to summon up the endurance, self-denial, and submission to guidance needed for a successful psycho-analysis, and necessary for the abandonment of certain conscious and subconscious aims.

However, as regards the origin of the development of social difficulties, we have to keep in mind the experimental sources in

[1] It is noteworthy that the stammerer has no difficulty in speaking in solitude. It is the conversation, the 'social aspect' of his speech, that creates a difficulty with which his constitutionally sensitive speech-centre cannot easily cope. And the only effective treatment for this disturbance is psychological.

[2] 'Social character' means the sum-total of ways of behaviour of an individual toward his fellowmen, and in communal life.

early childhood. I think the emergence of many misfits could be avoided by avoiding things which usually lead to a neurotic disposition. In this paragraph I have briefly mentioned a few points ; the reader is referred to Chapters VI and XXIV for further information on this problem.

6. Conscious and subconscious processes alike are engaged in dealing with the environment of the individual. And both spheres of the human mind are focused also on the individual's own ego.[1] A too accentuated attention toward one's own spheres of isolated existence is called introversion. The extravert is the true social being. As suggested above, the two spheres of consciousness work together to make a person an extravert or an introvert; yet we have to assume that the role of subconscious spheres in the introvert's attitude may, perhaps, be more substantial.

It is clear, however, that the environment, with its multifarious stimuli impinging upon the senses and the mind, constitutes a constant corrective against tendencies to introversion ; and it is a powerful incentive to the development and maintenance of the extravert attitude. What is called entertainment and diversion of the mind is, in fact, a planned intensification of this extraverting influence of the environment. There is no doubt that even the subconscious spheres are influenced by a diversion that appeals to the individual's taste ; and the subconscious, too, can acquire a change of accent from the autistic, i.e. self-centred, direction, into that of a better social adaptation.

7. Many of the readers of these chapters, which deal with different aspects of inter-human relationships, and which point to sources of difficulties and indicate possible ways of preventing them, may be interested in a brief discussion of the following problem. A considerable number of people, though uneducated and of no great natural intelligence, get on very well in life, and manage to keep on good terms with their fellowmen ; while just as many people who are well educated, and clearly conscious of the individual problems of social life, frequently experience difficulties and even shocking disappointments in the course of their social and family life, though they feel certain that they approach everything and everybody with the best intentions.

[1] Narcissistic factor.

Naturally, a healthy spontaneity of behaviour is the ideal of nature ; just as physical health exists when the organism works smoothly, without special attention being paid to it by the individual. Successful living is not meant to be experienced only by those who study life. A person who suffers frequently from indigestion, or who is a diabetic, and has therefore to acquire the detailed knowledge of bio-chemistry necessary for his dieting, is, in fact, rather at a disadvantage in comparison with the greater number of the ' happily ' ignorant. And people with accentuated psychological inclinations [1] are, if we may put it so bluntly, neurotics. They are those who feel, with too much self-awareness, the ' digestive process of their psyche ', and who, not infrequently, are lacking in that desirable automatism which exempts others from devoting special attention and energy to the accurate planning of their steps in life. More precisely, they are in fact deficient in social adaptation ; and their increased psychological inclination or analytically critical intellect, which at once sees the minute details of a phenomenon, is a kind of compensatory function of their mind. Yet this compensating talent seems, in most cases, insufficient to replace the healthy spontaneity of living.

Moreover, people of a complicated, differentiated mind mostly do not possess the faculty of understanding by empathy [2] the masses of less complicated people. The simple-minded individual can safely rely on what his feelings tell him. If he assumes in his fellowmen the operation of a similar outlook and taste, or pettiness, vanity, and selfishness, similar to what he experiences in his own mind, then he is more or less right in his assumption.

It is not incidental that people of such different types are in favour of a reformed and more socialized community. There are, apart from the great mass of poor and labouring people, a large number of ' original types '—scientists, artists (if they do not earn so much as to bias them), intellectual or sensitive personalities who cannot face disappointments, and no small number of other peculiar, solitary, unpractical people [3] ; in brief, all those who do not possess the healthy and unqualified spontaneity of thinking, feeling, and striving for practical aims. I do not doubt that many of these latter persons would indeed become more

[1] Looking at things from a psychological angle.

[2] Empathy is the process of feeling oneself into the fellowman—' putting oneself into his place '.

[3] The great number of ' good-for-nothings ' who swell the revolutionary crowds do not belong to the types here enumerated. They are ready to join any revolution, and hail any change that will enable them to take part in destruction and the creation of chaos, and to enjoy a short spell of idleness.

productive and more social, and consequently more healthy in their feelings, if they could be spared some of the pricks and handicaps that ensue upon the competitive system in economic and social life.

Many a man previously inefficient becomes active, persistent, productive, full of poise and courage, if put into an economic position or working conditions in which he can be more or less sure of justice and of due acknowledgment of his work, and in which he has to deal—whether as chief or subordinate—with people for whom logical argumentation, sincerity, and sense of duty represent the chief factors of their own life, and consequently, the foundations also of communal life.

Individuals of the ' sensitive ' or ' idealistic ' type, who are not quite capable of competing with the reckless behaviour of the others, tend to comfort themselves by contrasting their own refinement with the uncouthness and rudeness of the others, and then to withdraw into the life of splendid isolation, that is so much easier than battling with the world of painful realities. No little spiritual and scientific progress has originated from representatives of this sublimated and isolationist (autistic) [1] type of individuals. However, in scholastic education the praise of such over-refined attitudes should be rather limited ; and courage, and a little healthy indifference to the imperfections of human nature and behaviour, should be taught and developed by training. For the number of those who in their sheltered Olympian solitude develop into an original personality, or genius, is very small, and the number of those who merely become unfit for life is far greater. Individual sensitiveness should be treated with consideration, since a measure of latitude means for many people their only way of ease and happiness. But in the education of children, who are *not yet* beyond the hope of developing a sense and faculty for realities, and a toleration of unavoidable facts, unpleasant though they may be, the encouragement of a healthy, not over-sensitive average, and the fight against the feelings of weakness and inferiority, should be the main line of treatment. No true talent can be really frustrated in its development by such an education toward a healthy toleration of the cruder manifestations of life. That solitude of individualism, necessary for research and art, and for a meditative way of life, to which some person may feel attracted, enforces itself with their growing maturity. Any previous education toward realism and a less sensitive attitude cannot but have a beneficial effect on the

[1] The expression coined by Bleuler.

individual, and on his achievements in the fields of art, research, and the speculative sciences. The more deeply the individual personality is influenced by the *social process*, the more will his peculiar individuality, and the individual character of his output, mirror existing spiritual conditions. After all, effective adaptation stimulates in the deepest layers of the psyche the spirit of humanity, appreciation of one's fellow-beings, and devotion to the social community. And the art and science and philosophy springing from such a mental soil cannot but be more human than if developed on the soil of introverted isolation of the personality.

8. It may be useful briefly to survey the psychological factors operative in the individual in his capacity of a subordinate, carrying out his social contribution, and earning his living, as an employee. The first requisite is *a fair degree of subordination* to the guidance of another individual, or of other individuals. The ready subordination to an abstract factor—State, Society, Religion, etc.—is not necessarily paralleled by the faculty of easy subordination to a particular person who represents the abstract authority, or who is simply a superior economic or political factor. This latter kind of *personal adaptation* is greatly dependent on primitive mental functions that are beyond intellectual and intentional mental activity. There are mental structures deriving a certain satisfaction from the submissive situation [1] which sufficiently counter-balances the similarly natural tendency of ' revolting '. But doubtless many irritable personalities feel in any situation of subordination—however customary and even dignified—the element of attack on their freedom and personal value. Besides this nervous constitutional factor, the particular experiences during development in childhood and youth may determine the later attitude throughout life toward subordination. Individuals whose personality was practically broken by an educational pressure beyond their constitutional tolerance may later, in their occupational life, play the role of submissive, obedient, but certainly not impressive subordinates. Their yielding and collaborating attitude is easily shaken by any change in the social or political structure. They are those who swell the crowds of revolutionary masses—if the power of the previous regime is obviously reduced ; and they constitute also those masses who easily submit to, and collaborate

[1] Cf. (2), pp. 74-75.

with, any new ' boss ', no matter whether he is a more or a less humane and civilized social factor than the removed one.

Much depends on impressions retained by the youth about the past social position of his parents. Through the process of identification, the shortcomings from which the father had to suffer may induce the son to measure everything in society by those unpleasant impressions. For instance, any person earning more than the father of the individual in question used to attain is a ready object of envy or of a particularly keen criticism. And any degree of achievement of the son surpassing the career of his father may satisfy him, and this satisfaction may set undesirable limits to his aspirations.

If the father suffered conspicuously from economic limitations and social oppression, his offspring may become an irreconcilable enemy of all authority, of anybody who represents guiding and leading superiority. In a substantial number of individuals, however, the painful experiences of the past instil rather an increased readiness to collaborate and submit, in order to retain one's own social position surpassing the level of the parents. If the wielders of authority represent justice, and civilized aims and methods of work and organization, the above sources of readiness on the part of the subordinates may become irrelevant. The improved and appropriate conditions of their adult existence transform their neurotic character of subordination into a pleasant and free sense of collaboration. *In the individual of average psycho-nervous organization no past can be stronger than a fairly satisfactory present.* This holds good for the spheres of the individual's subjective life as well as for his faculty of extraversion, adaptation, and collaboration.

The number of individuals whose subconsciousness directly transfers their repressed resentment against the authority of their parents on to the superior in the course of their earning life is not, to judge by my analytical experience, so great as is usually assumed by psychological accounts in the past. This type exists undoubtedly. But, as may be seen from my exposition here and in Chapter XI (2),[1] the relationship between the subconscious attitude toward the parents and the general social behaviour of an individual is mostly not simply congruent, but greatly modified and complex.

A certain measure of identification with the aims of the employee is a further factor, necessary for successful subordination and co-ordination in employment. It is an everyday

[1] P. 58.

experience that the employees of a firm with principles of fairness, or of an administrative office with a guiding spirit of a higher quality, work readily and happily. However, individual types may gain substantial satisfaction from participating in corruption, exploitation, and suppression.; though they themselves occupy a totally insignificant and financially weak position. Such employment is one of the many modes of satisfying aggressive and base tendencies,[1] to which the person in question would not dare to subscribe openly in independent individual life. Hence, it can easily be understood that Governmental regimes of a non-democratic and non-socialistic character find ready employment for psychopaths, and find ready obedience from people who, psychologically judged, are semi-criminals. The authorities charged with the task of education and legislation still have insufficient knowledge and understanding of the true structure of the human psyche, and of the working conditions of subconscious processes. And accordingly, the valuation of educational principles, of the particular modes of behaviour of the citizen, and the whole problem of ethics and values, is, to a large part, guided by past errors and tentative or merely wishful conceptions, scholastic or religious.

The actual life of a generation and the theoretical knowledge of its scientists can never be entirely congruent. The best possible and most up-to-date reform of the principles guiding education, legislation, and jurisdiction could *not* eradicate deficiencies. But who dares to deny that at least the very principles of judgment, planning, and action, on the part of responsible authorities, ought to be attuned to established knowledge, in order *to avoid the avoidable and to increase the attainable*?

There is no exaggeration in saying that a substantial part of ethical, legal, and socially beneficial behaviour at present is due to the effect of neurotic motives, undignified attitudes, and avoidable oppression. Certainly, on the whole, the role of intelligent free collaboration and subordination in communal life is not greater than the part played by the before-mentioned factors. The difference between the two foundations is obvious. More intra-mental freedom implies more subjective satisfaction, and also a firmer quality of the ethical social order. That which is legally required and socially expedient is at the same time genuinely aimed at and liked by the individuals ; and they will not easily abandon the foundations of *their satisfactory social order.*

[1] Cf. Chs. IV and V.

CHAPTER XIV

PUBLIC SPIRIT AND THE STATE

It is inevitable for man, and it cannot be different, that his opinions and beliefs should be greatly influenced by external 'pressure', by suggestion, to which, fortunately, being a social and not a solitary being, he is everywhere subject. The individual's intellectual capacity is limited; just as one has to rely for most of what one needs for physical life on the productive capacity and the collaboration of others, so one is dependent on one's immediate environment, or on literary information, for a great part of one's knowledge, ideas, and judgments. Through the process of identification, so important for social life, the individual is able to share others' opinions, realizing, however, that he, by free choice, agrees with what they have found.

Why not utilize, in a planned manner, this socio-psychological fact? Why not put more emphasis on the creation of a more humane and more socially fit 'public opinion'? In many countries one is forced into being a patriot and a law-abiding citizen, both qualities which are certainly to be approved; though the factor of external force, applied for their attainment, may cast a shadow on their purity and higher value. Yet why grant so much 'individual freedom' to those who would, with the same readiness, be prepared to accept an elaborated social moral code? Why leave the field open to primitive or reckless demagogues, ignorant preachers of hatred and prejudice, without counteracting them by a more humane and scientific State-philosophy?

It might be replied that it is beneath the dignity of a Government to deal with such philosophical spheres of life; and also beneath the 'dignity of democracy' to interfere, even indirectly, with the freedom of thought of its citizens. *De minimis non curat lex.*

One cannot agree with this aloofness and generosity; since we have suffered so many untoward experiences of prejudice and of propaganda on a large scale in the distant and immediate past. If to have open prejudices really disqualified a man for 'public esteem', and at least for being in the direct employ of the State, many a man would exert more repression upon his neurotically distorted mind, and would try hard to make at least a show of the approved social outlook, the broad-minded intellectual attitude. The majority of these prejudiced people are not very brave, not very independent-minded—they share this weakness, unfortunately, with a great many well-intentioned individuals—and most of them give in very easily for the sake of expediency.

It is well known to the student of the social sciences that the valuation of goods is determined not only by their actual importance and usefulness. The general opinion, the general fashion, with regard to a certain commodity, may induce tens of thousands of people to find it useful and desirable, though without this factor of being in fashion they would never have done so. The same sociological phenomenon applies also to public opinion in general.

A Governmental system which tolerates the growth of private prejudice or hatred is not genuinely discharging its duty, or at least not sufficiently. Apart from indifference, there are two possible motives for the failure of Governments to exert more pressure against manifestations of hatred and of socially harmful prejudices. One motive will be, at least to some extent, consciously in the minds of some people with political power. Their argument runs as follows : " Let the people have their bit of aggressive pleasure ; let them enjoy their hatred and even a moderate exploitation of a certain group or stratum of the population ; in exchange for this they will be all the more ready to bear the burdens of public duties and political restrictions." This was once so in Egypt, where, according to the Bible[1] and to subsequent historical research, a new dynasty, being anxious about the consolidation of its freshly conquered supremacy, had created a special class of rightless people, on whom all the others could proudly look down as inferiors. By this method of ' abreaction ' —as psychologists call the process of finding satisfying substitutes for repressed tendencies—the hatred of the people was turned from the new dynasty and its followers against others, the ' Sons of Israel '.

The second motive that may underlie the aloofness of the governing groups with regard to ' humanitarian propaganda ' is something that belongs to the more subconscious spheres. We cannot expect people easily to believe it. It is the possible subconscious approval of aggressive tendencies. The individual may overcome any conscious approval, any inclination to take an active part, but his tendency may still not be sufficiently neutralized to prevent tacit enjoyment of the aggression perpetrated by others. Many ' tabooed ' things, according to psycho-analytical research and belief, can be approved and enjoyed subconsciously, under the disguise of apparent disinterestedness in all these

[1] Cf. Exodus.

matters. Let us point out this possibility to all those who wish to learn anything of the truth, even if its application to themselves may taste bitter.

A truly sincere lover of mankind, or a dutiful politician and leader, is never disinterested in, and never tolerant toward, the 'inferior types of public propaganda'. What would be thought of the medical profession if it refused to study the physiology of excretion because it is a 'low type' of activity? Apart from disregarding the abdominal diseases from which so many people suffer, the neglect of the whole problem of preventing the spread of typhoid and dysentery—to mention only something well known—would inevitably follow such a 'superclean' attitude. But that is the very thing that happened in the immediate past in political spheres. And this tolerant attitude actually increased the unspeakable misery of millions, who surely were not inferior in human value to those fortunate ones who stood inactive during the early spread of the social and cultural pestilence.

CHAPTER XV

CONTINUITY OF CONDITIONS AND TRADITIONALISM

1. The individual needs a certain constancy of conditions for his well-being, and no less so does the social organization. The injurious effect of a sudden change of the outside temperature on the general physical condition of man, or the indigestion arising from a sudden change in the customary diet, is illustrative of this phenomenon. The complicated physiological processes occurring within the body, building up and dissolving bio-chemical compounds, producing and regulating the body-temperature, distributing different stuffs to different organs according to their varying needs, are all destined to produce energy for the *various* activities; but at the same time to maintain a certain necessary *constancy* of chemical conditions within the individual cells. Similar requirements hold good for the mental life of man. His personality, the core and essence of his 'being', has to be maintained at any cost, in spite of the multitude of impressions and stimuli impinging upon it from without, and amidst the constant changes in his thinking, feeling, acting, and in his reacting to the events of his environment.

The subjective feeling of being fairly well balanced is, in fact, indicative of the needed objective ' constancy of the personality '. This inner constancy is the guarantee of, and the source of energy for, the efficient variability of the ' life-process ' in its fullest sense. A certain static condition of the psyche is the prerequisite of its dynamics.

And the case is similar with regard to social conditions. The individual cannot plan, cannot work, cannot feel at ease or as secure as he needs to be, if that which yesterday was white appears today to be black, and what seemed to be permanent and dependable proves overnight to be insubstantial, ephemeral, and deceptive. The continuous and multifarious activity and progress within society depend on the existence of a certain simultaneous constancy in it.

2. From the realization of this necessity follow the principle and practice of the continuity of the legal system of a country. If a new measure of reform has to be introduced, the first question is whether it fits into the existing legal system. No doubt this is a useful rule—provided that the basic principle of that legal system as a whole is social justice and the cause of humanity. In this case there is really no better guarantee for guarding the interests of the citizen than to see that any new measure remains consistent with the existing body of legal definitions and regulations. Yet, as with almost everything on earth, this very principle of legal continuity can also bear—and has borne on innumerable occasions—fruits which are poison to the general human well-being.

Similarly, a free Parliament for the nation and freedom of expression for the individual are certainly buttresses of a world with happy inhabitants. But only within limits ; we have seen this to be only too true. There is one fundamental mistake that can be made on this—to assume that freedom itself is the supreme intra-political aim of a State-community. In other fields of life we always subscribe to the corrective rider ; individual freedom, yes, but only in so far as it is not harmful to others, only in so far as it is really ethically beneficial and productive of happiness. In public affairs, both principles, the older one of legal continuity and the newer one of political freedom of the individual, have at times involved, and still threaten to involve, a certain measure of risk ; and, in fact, they have even proved in some degree obstructive of true and universal human progress.

3. Only one logical step could right the wrong, so far as is humanly possible. And that is *to make the greatest happiness of the greatest number of citizen-individuals, so far as reality permits, the supreme guiding principle of a modern State-organization.* And the carrying out of this task, so far as is possible under human conditions in our day, should be made the most serious duty of the whole administration.[1]

The natural and financial resources of a country at any particular historical period are given and limited. Its international political weight is dependent upon its own relative strength, and on its value and general significance to its neighbours. But beyond question, in spite of all these limitations, there is no country today that could not be rendered capable of far-reaching internal progress. There is no country and no Government that could not, with more venturesome spirit and more reforming initiative, give its own citizens at least twice as much ease and happiness as they have.

The natural tendency of inertia manifested in all physical and mental processes implies that to do more than in the past, or to act differently, would require more energy, increased attention, and a certain amount of self-denial. The public administrators, central and local, are human individuals. They may be, and frequently are, individuals of energy and ability above the average ; nevertheless, not all of them will refrain from enjoying the subjective advantages of more or less conservatism, and they might prefer to remain within the safe boundaries of legality and of existing conditions ; without even considering how to further the interests and increase the happiness of their fellow-citizens. It is hardly possible to expect from Civil Servants in general, whether in higher or lower positions, exceptional initiative and courage, to expect them to go out of their way in their autonomy, and to do for the public more than is required by the letter of the law, if not encouraged to do differently by some legal force or by public opinion ; that is, if they are not driven by their explicitly defined duty and by their personal interests.

There is no real obstacle to such a reformed State-idea. Only the misapplication of formal legal traditions, and the convenient compulsion of habit, may prevent its materialization. The manager of communal affairs, i.e. of the lives of the citizens, should be directed to keep to the letter of the regulations as long as the positive, i.e. human spirit of the law is being carried out. But it should be his right, and even his duty, to depart from the

[1] Cf. Jeremy Bentham's conception of State-duty.

letter of the law if, in a particular case, it appears obvious that only hardship and individual injustice would ensue from the application of a particular legal principle.

He should, of course, be able to give an account for his decision—an account that does not refer to some small paragraph of regulations but is based on the principles of a humane social science.

In individual life, too, it is only a physique and mind of a deficient type that cannot cope with new difficulties, and that keeps on with its unaltered habitual automatism, without even attempting to accommodate itself to a new situation, with the new measures it requires for self-preservation.

CHAPTER XVI

EXTERNALIZATION OF INNER PROCESSES. PARANOIA AND PREJUDICE

1. Paranoia is a very interesting type of psychosis (mental disease). The patient suffers from a delusional system, the content of which is, in different varieties, that he is an extraordinary individual, who is being envied or ' interfered with ', persecuted or even physically harmed, by a known or by a mysterious person or persons ; in most cases the suspicion refers to a whole organized body, in possession of extraordinary and even superhuman powers and resources as they pursue this aim of persecution. If the delusional belief stresses chiefly the experience of being persecuted, we speak of paranoia persecutoria.

Many persons, especially sensitive individuals with ambitions rather beyond their actual capabilities, or people who are too fond of overt appreciation, and who cannot easily bear the inevitable disappointments and pricks of social life, often feel that they are insufficiently appreciated, unjustly slighted, looked down upon, or even thwarted. In brief, they have mental experiences of the paranoid (paranoia-like) type, without, however, losing in essentials their sound common sense, which enables them still to carry on with life, and more or less to recognize that they may be carrying their resentment to excess, and to realize that they are not alone in having failures.

The psychotic patient is different. In his diseased mind [1]

[1] In the true uncomplicated paranoia, so far no examinable change of the brain-

there is no doubt that he, and he only, is right ; he feels certain that his belief in being persecuted and interfered with, in a manner and to a degree which to his normal fellowmen appears impossible and only 'imagined', is based on facts. The paranoiac may firmly believe that all the newspapers are bribed or otherwise induced to take part in a campaign against him ; and that the small advertisements contain hints about him ; he may also feel that people are 'misusing' his energies, by means of distant electric devices.

There is today [1] no doubt that the persecution felt by the paranoiac originates within the mind, and signifies an inner enemy ; it indicates some disturbance within his own mind which make him feel uneasy and as if threatened. Through externalization of this inner 'enemy' the mental disharmony is changed [2] into the interfering external world, i.e. the persecuting persons and their numerous torturing instruments, possible and impossible.

This process of externalizing the internal is not peculiar to the paranoiac psychosis. It is a universal human quality. We cannot help the fact that the human psyche is not as simple a structure as we should like it to be. We do not know why it is so, and why it cannot be less complicated ; why we have to carry in ourselves thoughts which are not conscious at all, and others which are not always capable of becoming conscious. We do not know why it is that so frequently we cannot make up our mind, cannot come to a clear decision, having the feeling of two or even more possible courses in connexion with the same thing. We do not know sufficiently why it is, or how it is, that love, and a little envy or resentment, can exist simultaneously in our minds toward the same person ; that, similarly, self-confidence, and the sure knowledge of our own value, has so frequently to be so intensely complicated by the simultaneous or alternating feeling of insufficiency of our self ; why we are a little insincere, even

cells or of the hormonal system has been discovered. In the schizophrenic type, however, there are some indications of tangible alterations of the brain and hormonal processes.

[1] The first analysis of paranoia was described by Freud in 1911.

[2] The environment is, in fact, the chief source of attacks on man's life. The savage, and also the primitive mind of all ages, has even blamed external magic influences for any intrinsically caused physical or mental distress. And perhaps there is much truth in this conception. It is possible that the human body and mind however weak in inborn constitution, owes its difficulties ultimately to the rough and 'hostile' physical environment and to the somewhat difficult claims of society. The paranoiac is consequently logical in carrying out in his mind the 'exchange' of causal conceptions. Freud made a subtle remark concerning the above problem. It appears, he said, as if the paranoiac 'sensed' the unconscious repressed aggressive tendencies in others.

when we intend to be most sincere ; a little selfish, and thinking of our own benefit, even if finally we decide to act, in the case in question, as pure altruists. It is a fact that there is nothing so complicated in the whole world, as far as we know, as the functioning and structure of the human psyche.

And our urge to libidinal satisfaction, and to the specific, erotically coloured, love for a fellow-being—how complex, how intricate a matter it is, even if not looked at through the magnifying apparatus of psycho-analysis. And now comes science, and states that this very human function is even more complex than we are wont to think it is. There is, for instance, a potential inclination in everybody to feel in a homosexual way. Indeed, immature, adolescent boys would with no difficulty be induced to a sexually coloured play with a playmate of the same sex. Only through the coming into play in adolescence of the overwhelming vital energy of the other, the so-called hetero-sexual tendency, does the homosexual one become pushed into latency and into the ' subconsciousness '. But on rare occasions, in the dream-world during sleep, one may experience peculiar scenes, inexplicable except through the knowledge of this background-homosexuality. The fact that each of us has in his blood-stream, to a minimal but still necessary degree, the sex-hormones peculiar to the opposite sex, dovetails into this phenomenon of emotional bi-sexuality.[1]

It was an apt observation by Freud, that several paranoiacs showed an over-emphasis of their subconscious homosexual complex. And his explanation was that the ' inner enemy ' which makes a number of such psychotic persons feel uneasy and threatened is their own accentuated subconscious homosexuality. Through externalizing this inner mental (intra-psychic) factor, and personifying it, the paranoiac patient feels as if he is being threatened by some kind of outside magic influence or by powerful enemies. Many of such paranoiac patients of another (the schizophrenic) group experience and state even that " people are tampering with their genitals " during their sleep, by distant X-rays, or similar far-reaching magic or ultra-modern devices.[2]

2. Externalization of inner psychic difficulties, ' personification '

[1] Folliculin (the female hormone) is always detectable in the urine of man. The first trace of this modern biological notion of basic bi-sexuality may be detected in the biblical conception about the creation of the woman from the body of the man—and in similar accounts in the myths of various races.

[2] However, there are other tendencies, complexes too, which are symbolized by the persecuting factor in paranoiac experience.

of intra-mental facts, is, as has been said, a process not peculiar only to the psychotic. The psychotic differs in this respect from the non-psychotic only in ' overdoing ' it, owing to a substantial disorder of his brain-function. The personification of inner mental processes occurs first of all in our dreams. A sleeping person may, by chance, have covered up his face with his pillow and feel an impediment in his breathing—and may subsequently have a dream about " two people fighting with each other fiercely until one suddenly jumps to the window, and violently throws it open in order to escape ", a not infrequent plastic dream-transformation of a person's difficulty in breathing during sleep. Or an individual feels in doubt whether to spend his hard-earned money to help his impoverished brother, or to buy for himself a car which he badly needs—and he may dream that " the rich Jewish business man is showing off with his savings, and refuses to sell his goods for a reasonable price to the dreamer, who is very annoyed about his meanness ". This latter instance, which I have chosen from my case-records, introduces us directly into our problem. In it the meanness of the dreamer himself is personified and shifted on to the ' Merchant of Venice '.

Not only in our dreams, but fairly frequently in daily life, we carry out such an externalization and projection of our innermost subconscious tendencies on to others in our immediate or distant surroundings. This process seems to be a kind of safety-valve of the mind, to get rid of uneasiness existing within the spheres of one's own psyche. The regularity and the great extent of this mode of ' emotional thinking ' in people of all kinds shows its significance, and indicates that there is an *inner necessity* for such a safety-valve. But the fact that, owing to this phenomenon, people too easily ascribe to others motives and characteristics of baseness and obnoxiousness, and this from a deep-seated subconscious tendency to do so, is a very serious one, and presents a very difficult social problem.

Before proceeding with the discussion of this phenomenon, however, I want to say a few words in excuse of the above. From the study of dreams, psycho-analysis has arrived at the conclusion that the shifting on to others of unethical tendencies of the individual is a kind of ' ethical improvement '. If, for instance, a sleeping person feels a slight toothache, he may succeed in shifting this untoward experience on to another person ; and he may dream that " Mr. So-and-so is racing to the dentist ". This probably makes the sleeper bear his pain more easily ; it is not he who has to suffer, and who next day will have to suffer still more. Similarly, the dreaming mind projects all tendencies which conflict with one's own morality, but which as elements of one's nature do nevertheless exist in one's own mind, on to another person. And this indicates a certain insight into the reprehensible character of the tendency. In the spheres of concrete activities, too, one often does something which one dislikes and even disapproves as being not quite fair, but which one feels obliged to do for one reason or another.

Now, the above mechanism or externalizing of one's inner uneasiness or inner hatred, or one's repressed sexual trends, on to others, obviously implies such a condemnation of the ' tabooed ' inclination. If one bears within oneself the tendency to aggression, hatred, destructiveness, to a substantial degree, or if, in one's deeper mental make-up, one is altogether lacking in pleasant, peaceful harmony, then the dim realization of all this is followed by its subconscious condemnation ; and then there emerges a counter-tendency to be rid of all that is disharmonizing the structure of the personality. This state creates the uneasiness which, in its turn, sets into motion the externalizing procedure. Subsequently, one feels that certain individuals, or, preferably, large groups, are not fair, not human, not cultured, not ethical enough to be acknowledged as equal and as human. They are base, dangerous, and deserving of contempt, hatred, and even active aggression. The purpose and the effect of such an externalization are double. First of all, the inner disharmony is, as it were, thrown out from one's own personal structure, and shifted on to others (projection) ; and then, all the fury of one's condemnation (in essence, a self-condemnation), one's distress about and fight against the condemned tendency, is put into operation ; and so the process of purification (subconsciously aimed at the purification of the self) is carried out at the expense of others. As if so the world, our internal and external world, of justice and ethics has been saved from the insidious menace of aggression or of perverse sexuality of others ; and in general from everything that disturbs and distorts human harmony.

3. It has already been briefly pointed out, in Chapter XI,[1] that there are individuals whose psycho-nervous constitution is unsatisfactory from birth, owing to early disturbances of development. It is not well fitted to deal with the continuous flow of subconscious processes, and not capable of maintaining a fair

[1] P. 64.

harmony within their mind. They are, more or less, always disharmonic. The vague awareness of their deepest disharmony stimulates various kinds of neurotic counter-measures, i.e. attempts at coping with their dysbalance. One mode of doing so is the extensive employment of externalization, as described above. And if there is also an accentuated inclination for producing hatred, then this aggressiveness, together with the process of externalization (projection), leads to an unceasing desire to accuse and to attack, to despise and to hate others, that is, to cherish prejudice.

It is very probable that one important source of the easy creation of hatred is the dissatisfaction with one's own disordered and insufficient subconscious structure. It is as if one hated oneself, revolted against that unknown agent responsible for one's inner disharmony. This, however, is for most cases a more or less theoretical interpretation.[1] But in medical practice one not infrequently meets people who, when they have to bear some minor discomfort due to their own nervous debility, fly into a temper and rail at fate or at their parents for having brought them into such a difficult life. Accordingly, it is quite probable that a person may develop unmotivated hatred, owing to his general constitutional nervous disharmony. We shall see later [2] that this interpretation can be supported by an interesting observation which I was able to make in a number of cases during careful psycho-analysis.

The upshot of what has been said so far on the process of externalization and on its employment in creating prejudice for 'abreacting' [3] hatred, is that a neurotic emotional urge (parapathic process) is at work in both cases, in the general process of projection and in that of cherishing prejudice and political or racial hatred. This is today the accepted scientific theory on this matter.

Bleuler, the greatest psychiatrist of his age, following Kraepelin aptly remarked that the first condition for producing psychotic delusions is a peculiar mental need in the individual for having these, on the face of it unpleasant delusions. But just

[1] A young man, previous to his treatment, could not work in a team or under supervision of a manager, since he always felt embarrassed and imagined that he was being ridiculed by his employers or fellow-workers. In the course of his psycho-analysis he realized that he was externalizing his inner conflicts, and that his morbid feelings were due to his innate psychopathic difficulties, the latent and 'qualified' inheritance from his manifestly psychotic father. Later he sometimes admitted: "*I hate all people who may see my nervous embarrassment, because they may think that I am 'soft'. I could even kill them.*"

[2] Ch. XVIII.

[3] Giving vent to a feeling with subsequent relief.

the same applies, as we have seen, with regard to externalization and prejudicial hatred. The prejudiced individual needs, for his mental process, those others on to whom he projects his inner disharmony. He could not live, as it were, without the existence of his existing or imagined adversaries, near or remote.

4. At the same time, it must be pointed out that it is the particular social condition, that social process so frequently referred to in this work, that enables and encourages the individual, in developing a certain prejudice, or even perhaps anti-social, anti-human attitudes, to cope with his innermost weakness and disharmony. If society and State would suppress by legal force, or by a strong public opinion, the development of such psycho-neurotic manifestations, they would surely not come to the fore so abundantly. The same is the case with other neurotic trends, as mentioned on p. 65. If, for instance, the hoarding of money had not a certain social significance in the life of 'normals', the pathological thriftiness, as a neurotic trend, would have no meaning for the individual. A great many neurotic character-traits are beyond understanding except as distortions of existing social phenomena. For instance, social morality is keenly interested in the regulation of sex. Marriage, the concept of monogamy and fidelity, a certain shyness and self-restriction in respect of sexual emotions, all these are meant to safeguard a reasonable measure of order and peace among people. But the individual psyche frequently employs a self-restriction going far beyond the demands of social morality. If the subconsciousness aims at the fulfilment of sexual tendencies which are not tolerated by the inner moral laws of the same individual, for instance, if incestuous, homosexual, or polygamous tendencies menace the harmony of the subconscious spheres, then in response to all these impulses there may ensue a neurotic disturbance of the sexual functions such as sexual frigidity, impotency, fear of sexuality, and so on. Or if a person feels deep down that his marriage would very much hurt his parents, or interfere with his own emotional fixation on his parents, then his psycho-nervous system may easily solve the problem without any contribution from his conscious intellect. It may create a disturbance of his sexual faculty, and so prevent him from marriage. It is clear that these symptoms are neurotic copies of the existing normal social limitations on sex.

And similarly, many unpleasant character-traits are essentially the outcome in distorted forms of approved social attitudes.

Competitiveness in business, art, science, politics is part of our social life. But if one thinks of the many unpleasant and socially harmful manifestations of ruthless competitiveness, vanity, striving for prestige, etc., one hardly recognizes in them the direct influence of approved principles of social life.

To recapitulate and sum up : It is certain that the manifestation of prejudice and hatred, and its organization on the scale customary not only in our times but throughout social history, is made possible only by the social process. We do not know exactly what would happen if the social process did suppress these particular anti-social neurotic manifestations ; we do not know how men's minds would then 'abreact' their disharmony. But such a social experiment is worth while. The present writer thinks that under such social conditions the neurotic dysbalance of the individual might be less altogether. First of all, because a sincere fight of the community against prejudice could not remain an isolated reform, but could only be part of a more general improvement. But secondly, we know from educational psychology that the creation of certain neurotic, over-compensating character-traits can be successfully suppressed without real harm to the individual.

The process of externalization is, however, not always aggressive in character. It may be just of the opposite type. If people too readily think, for instance, that others do not appreciate them, or even that they despise them, or fail to understand them, then this is, similarly, only an externalization of their own dissatisfaction with themselves. The underlying idea is : "I do not find myself worthy to be appreciated and to be considered as the equal of others." Or : "If people knew how self-centred or selfish or incapable of loving others I am, then they would not appreciate me." The third possible background for such ideas may be the fact that these people, by dint of their innate nature, wish for too much love, and too much appreciation beyond what is normal and justified for them to claim ; but instead of realizing their exaggerated claims, they project the wrong, the deficiency, on to others.

Probably, however, under better social conditions much subconscious disharmony, even of the constitutional type, could be converted into the desire for more productivity, such as many people do spontaneously reveal. The vague realization of their inner inefficiency stimulates these people to increased external activity and achievement ; a useful type of over-compensation (Adler).

CHAPTER XVII

AN INTERESTING CASE OF PARANOIA[1]

I PROPOSE now to describe an interesting case of paranoia which I had the opportunity to observe over a period of five years. I think it is a case of more than individual interest. The reader will see later why I am introducing this description as of illustrative significance, and why I am giving its analysis a substantial space in this volume devoted to the broader field of social psychology.

The patient was 51 years of age when she was brought to me by her husband. Her complaints were sleeplessness and general nervousness. Her husband supplemented her story by saying that " she imagines that people are speaking slanderously about her, though there is no truth at all in it ; it is just her imagination ". A typical case of persecutory paranoia. The husband added that the condition started a year earlier, a few weeks after his wife had suffered from an inflammation of her cheek (erysipelas). It happens not infrequently that people who have the constitutional inclination to develop a psychosis do so finally after some incidental infection, which, by temporarily upsetting the balance of health, however slightly, may pave the way for a mental illness which may have been already present, even in its particular structure, though not yet manifested. No doubt this woman was, even in her normal years, a kind of eccentric. She liked solitude, had no capacity for carefree merriment, and lived solely for her occupation—she was a teacher at a Roman Catholic school—and for her household. Her husband, a more natural fellow, was a teacher at the same school. They lived with his mother, who was in charge of the house, and who was a rather simple, uneducated, but quiet type of woman.

After I had had the opportunity of speaking to the patient three times, she told me more about her delusions. She thought that people wanted to alienate her husband from her, wanted her to be lowered in his esteem—and all this, so she said, had been planned and carried out by Jews. She firmly stated that if she only knew them, or the ringleaders, she would certainly kill them, since she was unable to go on living under such a constant strain. She admitted that she did not know why these people should be interested in such manœuvres against her, and—very interesting to hear—that she had never in her life spoken privately to a person of the Jewish race.

[1] The author is authorised to publish this case.

If she went through the street the passers-by said things, as for instance, " I do not know where she gets money from ", or " I think she is not quite well " : briefly, anything said about female persons that she happened to overhear, she applied in the true paranoiac manner to herself—and interpreted it in a slighting sense.

A proper analytical treatment proved impossible, since my patient was unable to supply the elementary prerequisite of such analysis, the detailed description of her life-story. It was certain only that she had been brought up in a family where the father was the supreme authority, and where there was not much spontaneity or merriment, only industrious study, courtesy, and the conventional occasions for a smile. During six months of attempted analysis she produced only three brief dream-recollections ; all of them connecting up with the memory of a trip she had made twenty-five years earlier to what is now the Italian Tyrol—a trip with her sister (who had remained a spinster) and with a gentleman who had shared their walks in the forests and their mountain-climbing.[1]

In her scanty recollections there was a frequent reference to an operation she had gone through seven years before her paranoia developed ; a polyp of the anal region had been removed under an anaesthetic. The analyst Stekel always stated that the subconscious of certain psychologically unstable people may construct, during such an operation, an imagined psychic trauma,[2] with the subsequent formation of a neurosis. I take it as probable that a similar process had taken place in my patient, and had become operative only later, during her fully developed paranoia ; for which, however, there had always been an inborn inclination of her personality-type.

She knew very well that I am a Jew, and that a great many of my private visitors, whom she had ample opportunities to see, were Jews. However, with unbroken confidence and obvious attachment she continued visiting me. On these occasions she began by making the usual complaints of persecutions and slights, and then regularly switched over to different physical complaints, for which she received from me either minor advice or harmless prescriptions. There was soon an obvious improvement in her condition : she became more sociable, and above all, she was able to carry out her duties at school, and tried to overlook the ' slights '. We call this process ' dissimulation ', since the patient is advised to pretend to be well and normal. She

[1] A clear symbol for the dream-analyst.
[2] A shocking experience, frequently of a sexual nature.

frequently even admitted the possibility of my suggestion that a great many of the utterances she heard might not have applied to her. Her essential paranoiac belief, naturally, did not change, since there was not even an attempt at proper analysis in her case. (Several analysts have succeeded a few times in their career in improving by analysis milder cases of paranoia.)

One day something happened which gave an interesting turn to the whole behaviour of my patient. Her husband, who had suffered for years from asthma and bronchitis, suddenly died from heart weakness. Now it came out that her husband had 'left her'; and I was also rather disturbed because the physician whom he had been attending for a number of years was a Jew; he had attended the patient until the last moment. After I heard that the funeral had taken place, I ventured a friendly call—and my patient seemed to be very composed, and pleased at my call. She also expressed her wish to continue with her half-hourly visits, three times a week—everything as in the past.

She came; and soon, with a smile, she confided to me her new secret. Her husband had not died, all that was only pretence, a fake funeral. A new teacher had been appointed to fill her husband's place at the school—and she thought that he was either a messenger from her husband, or even her husband himself, returning to her under a disguise. She decided soon for this second explanation; she only expressed her great embarrassment about this mystery, the possible reasons of which, she said, she could not even guess.

And now a remarkable thing regularly happened. Three times a week she visited her husband's grave, cared for the flowers and the tombstone, and then came straight away from the cemetery to me. The first part of the time was filled with a description of the state of the grave, the flowers, the careless gardener, the expenses—and then suddenly all this was not reality any more; she talked of her husband, "who is alive and is only awaiting the opportunity to cast off the spell forced upon him by mysterious people", amongst them a few Jews, strangers to her. I have to stress that, apart from her delusion, her behaviour was entirely rational, even, as described, in respect of her dead husband.

Apparently she was living simultaneously in two worlds. Or, alternatively—and this is my interpretation, which I advanced a long time ago for paranoia [1]—*her mind knew 'deep down' that all the persecution-business was only a symbol for a complex, i.e. for a different, emotionally charged idea. And, consequently, she could safely speak and*

[1] In *Psycho-analyt. Praxis*, 1932.

act in a way that proved her knowledge of the actual death of her husband. There was no essential contradiction in her behaviour. There also occurred another change; step by step she dropped the idea of persecuting Jews, and began to be impatient, even accusing her husband of reluctance to return to her.

Her condition gradually deteriorated, and she had to retire, but she remained attached to me until the last moment of my stay in Czechoslovakia, though she was of German nationality, read only the one German paper—already of the new type—available in the town, and was a very pious and devoted Roman Catholic, factors which, at that time, induced thousands to fall in with aggressive anti-Jewish behaviour. I even did not dare to tell her that I was leaving, perhaps for ever. I was at that time her only real support and friend, though she had her sister and mother-in-law; they frequently used to visit her, but of course did not understand her.

I submit this short description to my psychiatrist colleagues, and to all interested in the psychology of racial, religious, and general prejudice.

And now I should like to add a few words of explanation and interpretation. We are today convinced that all the symptoms appearing in neuroses, or in delusions of psychoses,[1] are only distortions of normal contents of the subconscious spheres. Or, to put it differently, symptoms have taught us a great deal about the probable processes of the normal subconsciousness. If I may use a very simple analogy—a tear in an elegantly tailored suit may allow the lining to become visible, and will then remind the onlooker that his suit—still a good suit—has the same quality of second layer, though well covered up. The relationship of subconscious mechanisms to the conscious and overt manifestations of the mind are of much the same type as the relations of the complicated set of wheels and springs and studs of the clockwork to the visible face and hands and figures.

The chief reason for my presenting this case in this volume is to illustrate the symbolic character of prejudices and the projection of inner complexes into resentment, hatred, and the idea of being threatened or persecuted. This illustration is, however, valid only if the thesis just mentioned is fact; that is, that neurotic and psychotic processes are essentially only distortions of normal intra-psychic events. And such pathological phe-

[1] It is only the 'content' that shows similarity in neurosis and psychosis respectively. The essence of the two processes is different. They are *not* as the layman thinks, and fears—different degrees of the same abnormality.

nomenon may be initiated through different causes—physical or mental shocks—producing such a ' tear ' in the integrity of the mind.

As to the peculiar picture in the above case, I should like to state that, to a substantial degree, it was expressive of my patient's regret at having married her husband, the son of such a simple mother. Anybody who decides on such a step in his life has subconsciously to face a process of adaptation. Traces of such an inner conflict and effort may become manifest, and the existence of such a not quite successful repression may even be one of the factors contributing to the gradual weakening of the emotion-self, or even—as in psychosis—of the intellect.

Jews, freemasons, and other socially tabooed groups, have been in the past a favourite object of externalization in delusional formations, as can be seen from contemporary textbooks.[1] But in the present case there was an additional factor which may have contributed to this subconscious choice of delusion. The mother-in-law of the patient, a very simple woman, used to tell her about the jewellery and furs of ' rich Jewesses ' which were deposited in the cloakroom of the opera house where she was for many years employed. This vexed my patient very much ; she was particularly vexed about the inferior occupation of her mother-in-law, and the Jew-motive may have been aptly expressive of her contempt both for her mother-in-law and for her husband. The translation of her delusion into the language of interpretation runs : " There is in my subconsciousness a burning hatred for my mother-in-law and contempt for her son, who is more attached to her than to me. I should not have married him." This idea was naturally ' alien ' to her conscience and her conscious mind, and after having been repressed it reappeared in the form of delusions, expressing her own idea in the form of accusations and persecutions from the outside (externalization).

CHAPTER XVIII

AN OBSERVATION OF THE PSYCHO-ANALYST

THE psycho-analyst is afforded the opportunity of closely examining the deeper mentality of people of considerable variety. True, they belong—apart from his colleagues in ' training

[1] In Continental countries.

analysis '[1]—to the type of personality that develops a neurosis in response to inner conflicts. The large number of manifest aggressors and dangerous haters rarely expose themselves to the searchlight of deep psycho-analysis. And, accordingly, the following observation, the significance of which the writer wishes to emphasize, is open from the very start to one possible objection, i.e. it is limited and one-sided in its sources.

There are people enough who are more or less anti-Semitic in their sentiments, and who miss no occasion to give expression to their anti-Semitism, or to let their particular actions be influenced by this widespread prejudice. There are, consequently, patients who would never visit a Jewish psychiatrist. Yet the conditions of the social structure in Europe have resulted in a disproportionately large number of Jewish doctors feeling the desire to take up this special field of research and of medical activity. The reason for this is complex : it is evidently based more or less on a special ' mental inclination '. As is well known, Sigmund Freud, William Stekel, Alfred Adler, and not a small number of other renowned writers on analytical psychology and successful psycho-therapists, were and are of Jewish origin. And the belief in the skill of a certain physician pushes into the background the anti-Semitic prejudice in a great number of patients. Now, people have no idea in advance, and fortunately so, about the method of free association. If they had, they would not so readily submit to analytical treatment. In the course of free associations all studied attitudes have to recede into the background. Thoughts, opinions, and emotions are freely expressed without consideration for absolute logic, convention, or moral sentiment. Such free associations are indispensable to analysis. And the analysed person has to learn to overcome the natural inhibition against this method of free, non-regulated expression of ideas which present themselves to his mind. Sentiments concerning the person of the analyst are not excepted. On the contrary ; for a very important technical reason, they have a first-class significance, being indicative of the so-called transference. If, then, the patient feels that he hates, at a certain moment, his analyst, or wishes to ' throw something at him ', or alternatively, if he feels that he loves or admires the analyst, and would like to share his private life, etc.—all these ideas have to be frankly expressed.

It is clear that the incidental anti-Semitic attitudes of the patient may also come upon the scene. After a time the patient learns to express them frankly, knowing that the analyst accepts

[1] It is necessary for a would-be analyst to undergo first a psycho-analysis himself.

such utterances with the same objectivity as expressions of love and admiration, by which he must not feel personally complimented.

The analyst knows that the greatest part of that which is felt by the patient about him is only transferred from other persons significant in the patient's past. It is mostly subconscious attitudes that are being transferred to the analyst ; for instance, repressed resentment or repressed love toward certain persons, mostly near relatives. This transference is the most important factor in psycho-analysis ; since as long as such transference-emotions are manifest, the substantial role of repressed tendencies is certain.

Anti-Semitism is not a repressed tendency, and consequently I think it is easy for the patient of a Jewish analyst intentionally to eliminate hating him from anti-Semitic tendencies—to make him an ' exceptional Jew '. The main emotional background of the patient's attitude toward him springs from subconscious, more or less repressed, sentiments. This is probably the chief reason why the analysis and successful treatment by a Jewish physician of people of even strong anti-Semitic tendencies in actual life is possible, apart from very few cases, in which the patient breaks off treatment at the very outset on some pretext.

Yet the free associations contain not only subconscious, i.e. forgotten, material, but, abundantly, all elements related to the likes and dislikes of the analysed individual. And here comes the observation to which I should like to draw the serious attention of psychologists and social research workers. The ' anti-Semitic ' free associations become fewer and fewer during treatment ; in most cases they do not occupy much time from the very start. Deep down there is no genuine anti-Semitism in our patients. As long as they are permitted to pour out their hatred against those who, in fact, did limit their life and pleasures, as long as they are permitted to describe in detail their genuine problems, conflicts closely touching their personality, they seem to have no interest in anti-Semitism ; though before treatment—and probably after the treatment has been finished—this attitude was, and will be again, manifest. I take naturally into consideration that the patient's anti-Semitism may disappear for the time of the analysis, for the sake of the Jewish analyst (there is naturally not the slightest interference on the part of the analyst with this tendency). But this cannot be simply a polite gesture or an intentional act of the mind ; such tendencies would still emerge, both in the free associations and in the dreams, if they possessed a sufficient emotional charge. I refer to what has been said above, about the sometimes violent expressions of hatred and contempt, as signs of transference, which are apparently directed against the analyst.

There is, for me, no other possible conclusion and explanation than to state once again that, deep down, only very few people are anti-Semites ; or, alternatively, that if people have another way of ' abreacting ' their hatred and other tabooed complexes, they do not need anti-Semitism ; especially if the analyst is a Jew, and the display of such a tendency would not particularly please him.[1] I venture to claim, after having been an analyst for fifteen years—and for ten years in a town where there was no Gentile physician practising psycho-analysis—that my observation is more or less worthy of attention.

A few of my colleagues whom I have had the opportunity to ask about this observation agree that anti-Semitic tendencies only very rarely constitute the content of free associations. The present author, therefore, simply submits his observation to all who are interested in the problem ; without, however, assigning too much practical significance to it and to his conclusions, so long as there is no opportunity of investigating the matter more closely, and with the collaboration of a larger number of psychologists in medical practice.

CHAPTER XIX

THE POLITICAL MIND

THE ' political inclination ' of modern man merits a special analysis. It cannot be denied that the institution of a free Parliament, with freely organized opposing parties, represents a marked progress in man's culture and social history. Yet, at the same time, we have learnt all too well the possible adverse aspects of the same institution. First of all, it is no secret that the general well-being of the masses is by no means sufficiently safeguarded by a free Parliament alone. Those who are in favour of a privileged class, or simply attached to unmodern traditionalism, have similarly their free party-representation ; and, owing to their usually greater opportunities of exerting influence, in the past they largely succeeded in their aims—more than was really

[1] In the social application : If the State and public opinion were displeased by anti-Semitic or similar reactions, they would not come easily into being.

beneficial for the nation, if this expression means the 'people' with their human needs. What I want, however, chiefly to stress here, is the intrinsic disintegrating function of such unlimited free political activity. Individualism is always ready to play its part—simply for the sake of the play itself—and by no means all individual likings and all party organizations are based on the foundation of truly beneficial social progress.

When speaking on the psycho-analysis of political activity, we must not forget that essentially we can only attempt a psychological 'explanation' of this phenomenon. Such an explanation may be superficial or deeper-going, and may be approaching the core of the truth, or only touching its periphery. Many, perhaps most, of psychological presentations of social phenomena are of a subjective, merely 'explanatory' kind. And, unfortunately, any social theory that does not succeed in touching upon the essence of the problem in question must absolutely fail to have sufficient influence on the minds of those engaged in social work and reconstruction, and must fail to affect the factual evolution.

The individual psycho-analyst is in the possession of experience of a very limited scope. He may analyse a smaller or greater number of individuals, but during his highly specialized professional work he hardly pays attention to those aspects of the personality which do not closely concern the neurotic conflict. However, the present author happened in the past to have had several patients actively engaged in party politics ; and since he has always been interested in the psychology of social phenomena, he did on occasion pay special attention to this aspect too. He is enabled to describe his impressions from his—admittedly very limited—experience on this point:

I myself feel surprise in reviewing the material, because it is clear that the particular political conviction and fierce interest of my patients in politics was, in most cases, very much in the background during their analysis. True, the chief interest during treatment is in personal health, and in the closer personal relations of the individual. But that is the very point I should like to state. It appears as if the 'political mind' of the individual does not connect closely with those deeper mental spheres with which the analyst is called upon to deal. I feel certain that in most cases fierce political convictions of people are not based on their genuine spontaneity. This is, in fact, to be expected, since the very existence of certain parties, and all the propaganda connected with them, are the chief factors in determining the adherence of many individuals to a particular political party. (Cf. p. 137.)

No doubt the membership of a particular political movement in our times is primarily devoted to concrete fights for concrete advantages. But as to the general tendency to create and to belong to parties, the central factor, so far as I can see in my cases, has been the ' exclusion of the others ', has been an attacking attitude. The building of groups, from which the great mass of the others, the ' heretics ', are to be excluded, seems the essentially significant and the fundamentally satisfying factor. True, party propaganda as a rule pretends to aim at the ultimate *inclusion of all* into its own organization ; and to make all adherents of its ' ideology '. Yet, if such universal acceptance of that party ideology were suddenly to take place, it is easy to foresee that, without some forceful, external preservation of the party unity, this unity would fairly quickly cease to exist. The members would miss the deeper satisfaction resulting from ' excommunication of the heretics '.

Doubtless any substantially improved social organization, and its scientific institutions, should discourage that kind of political sentiment and activity. If, however, groups of people were to vie with each other in solving the problems of how to increase social justice, and how to provide still better ways of attaining happiness, then the accent of their various group-buildings would be shifted toward the common aims, and only the methods of approach to such aims would be different. There would still be scope enough for satisfying the pugnacious, competitive party tendency ; for satisfying primitive claims to superiority because of the possession of the ' truth ' ; for enjoying not less primitively and more or less admittedly the fact that there are ' outsiders ' who are a little ' inferior ' in their fashion of grasping the ' right ' ways and means. But, on the whole, this mode of competition would lead to a better exploration of the social truth in its different aspects. The case is similar in the exact sciences and in chemistry and medicine. No doubt, personal ambition plays here, too, a very substantial role. And the creation of ' schools ', and of homogeneous scientific circles, is similarly facilitated by the ' clannish ' aggressive tendencies described above. Yet, on the whole, the outcome of competition in these scientific fields has always been some progress toward the common aim, the comfort and health of humanity. But the aims, the actual ultimate aims, of our political parties are from the very outset essentially different, and therefore their activity entails at least as much curse as blessing.

A social philosophy in which universal well-being is the

supreme principle, and a practical management of State affairs, based on such a foundation, fed by such a spiritual background and incentive, should automatically be followed, sooner or later, by a spontaneous collapse of the desire of people to engage in 'politics' in today's sense of the word. Such a universal and total collapse of political tendencies is naturally only a Utopian idea, projecting into the infinite future the gradual progress of true cultural improvement. But certainly, all the feverish political restlessness in Europe after 1918 was only a symptom of illness, the precursor of present events, the indicator of gravely unsatisfactory conditions.

And in this sense it may be stated that any substantial progress in social happiness, in mutual goodwill, based on an altered conception of human aims, and on an improved conception of State-organization, will inevitably be followed by a decrease of 'political activity'. What was in the past a characteristic of enslaved masses, their lack of interest in politics, may be in the future a sign of an intellectual superiority, finding no great interest in such a 'petty' occupation. To the psychologically minded onlooker, especially after he had attained a certain settledness of his own mind, and after having seen what occurs, in fact, in the depths of human nature, many a political fight may appear somewhat infantile. Certainly, so the psychologist dares to think, a game of tennis, played in the open, and out of the healthy spontaneity of the psyche, represents a more worthy interest for civilized man. The psychologist wants, however, to stress that in his negative criticism he has not in mind the perennially necessary struggles carried out through political activity, which truly aim at the cure of the many social ills.

There is a probability that an increased sense for problems of science, in so far as the latter aims at the decrease of human suffering and the increase of the enjoyable factors of life, may be able to replace much of the political tendency. Let us not forget that between the political interests of today and the political interests of long past centuries there is fortunately a great gap. Throughout history, almost all over the world, general interest and clashes were mainly concerned with prestige, accumulation of resources, religious conceptions, and, at the best, speculative scientific principles. The social problem, tackled by means of the empirical sciences and of psychological research, has never, until the last few decades, occupied men's minds in any substantial degree.

CHAPTER XX

THE STRANGER AND HIS ENVIRONMENT

1. Today, more than ever before, the problem of the ' stranger in a strange land ' merits the attention of the social psychologist. Whilst, in the past, emigration and immigration was more or less a problem limited to few individuals and chiefly concerning the emigrant, the stranger himself has now become, on the one hand, a phenomenon concerning tens of thousands, and on the other a particular problem for all the countries of immigration. What I am concerned to point out is that there exists a serious psychological problem of the environment of the stranger. There can be no question that the acceptance of the stranger may be, for some individuals and under particular conditions, a much more difficult task than is the adaptation of the stranger to his new environment.

It appears that the ' digestion of the new ' and the toleration of a stranger is a special task, with which not everybody is equally fitted to cope. The perception and elaboration of every new impression is certainly connected with a special effort of the mind. Whilst the majority of people feel stimulated by new impressions, a not inconsiderable number feel more or less disturbed, and dislike the stimulation coming from the new (neophobia). There are not a few people who dislike new dresses, a new kind of food, or books and papers different from what they are used to. The reluctance of this group throws, in fact, a certain light on what happens in the mind of everybody who is faced with something new. There must be brought into operation within the mind an adaptive process which is experienced by the mentally more alert and unburdened as stimulation, and by the reverse type as mental difficulty, resulting in the feeling of reluctance.

The general mass of our fellowmen are a potential source either of help and pleasure, or of competition and restriction. The number of those from whom the individual expects pleasure and advantage is limited ; whilst the far greater part of the ' others ' are members of that social community, the regard for which enforces the adaptive and self-restrictive, i.e. tolerant ' social ' attitude. The appearance of a stranger on the stage of communal life makes for a weakening of this adaptive attitude. The very fact of his ' being a stranger ', an individual with fewer legal rights and less backing than the others, automatically decreases the habitual sentiment of regard in the masses, and stimulates the emergence of that primitive attitude of intolerance which is always present, though in various degrees, behind the façade of the developed social tolerance. This process of shaking the foundations of social tolerance is naturally furthered by the difficulty, in the minds of many people, in coping with the new, as suggested above.

The average individual has attained a certain degree of social tolerance toward his fellow-countrymen. The newcomer, the stranger, constitutes an additional problem for his faculty of repressing hatred, aggression, and envy. Human sympathy in general, and an exceptionally pleasant impression created by the stranger, may decide the intra-psychic process in favour of additional tolerance. But how small is the number of those who are in possession of such exceptional charm as to please adequately all those whom—as strangers or as persecuted refugees—they have the opportunity to meet.

Humanity and the customary degree of sympathy may be insufficient to overcome the antagonistic attitudes described above. And, in addition to the factors mentioned so far, there is another one to be considered. I have pointed out already, whilst discussing the phenomenon of externalization, that people project their innermost complexes on to others. A similar process of projection may occur in the mind of the individual who meets a stranger. The latter becomes, by the very fact of his being different in language, appearance, and habits, a subconscious reminder and symbol of that which is ' strange ' within the individual, and he may be a welcomed object of the ' hating externalization '.

The single stranger, being hardly a factual competitor for many, can easily be assimilated by a multitude of people. It is as if his existence and his share in the means of life were divided among all the thousands of his environment, and found by the subconsciousness of these thousands as not substantial enough to harm them, and therefore negligible. All that remains manifest in their minds is the realization of his being something new, either interesting, or inferior, peculiar, an object of momentary entertainment and nothing else.

The social process, which in this case is essentially the particular attitude of the Government and political leaders, has naturally a marked influence on the reactions toward the stranger. There is nothing that influences the average person's social attitude more than the official backing, much or little, received by an individual on emerging as a new social element, without firm roots in the soil of the community. There is hardly a factor more substantial in modifying the reactions of an average person toward others in general than the amount of 'human position', that is, of individual or rather social prestige, enjoyed by these others.

2. There is, however, a peculiar factor, springing in the main from 'neurotic sources' in the mind of the environmental individual, which may make the social position of the stranger easier. And that is the not infrequent prejudiced attitude of people against their own countrymen. There is, naturally, in every life more or less frustration and disappointment. And the more closely related is the person responsible for the disappointment, the greater is the resentment in the mind of the sufferer. Repressed hatred against relatives may, through the medium of generalization, be projected on to one's fellow-countrymen, and may lead to that well-known attitude which sees in, and hopes from, anything foreign something superior, attractive, and desirable. This is especially obvious in the case of a foreign musician, writer, physician, clergyman; in brief, with persons who, by virtue of their particular occupation, appeal to the more intimate and higher psychic needs of their fellowmen. The subconscious formula of this 'apostasy' runs: "I shall love and appreciate the foreigner, because he is so different from those who are near to me, but who have disappointed me by not giving me their utmost attention and love."

Incidentally, the individual foreigner may be a skilled and useful person. He may bring something new into the sphere of the accustomed. And if he is in employment, he may naturally make added efforts to please his employer because of his *a priori* weaker position. Yet, as has been said above, that spirit of emotional antagonism toward those who are closer to one, that resentful and revengeful attitude, may meet the stranger half-way in his effort to strike root in the social soil of his new land of domicile.

We know this mental process from psycho-pathology; it is called differentiation of oneself—as a rule, from one's parents. It is one of the possible responses of the mind to difficulties as suggested in Chapter VI. If the child feels that he has not gained the necessary harmonious attitude toward his parents, because he feels that he has gone short of their loving attention, or because the child feels that his parents are not up to his own expectation in intellect, or morality, then there may ensue a tendency to be different, to be even of the utterly opposite kind. In the past, when Socialism was considered something inferior, many a young man felt attached to this movement from subconscious antagonism toward his capitalist father. And not infrequently the sons of strictly religious fathers are 'active' atheists. Were they only disinterested in religion, their attitude would be less militant and more tolerant.

A too accentuated, positive fixation to parents, but especially to the mother, may lead, through the medium of counter-regulation, to a similar tendency of differentiation. Such a man likes only women different from his mother; and he may also try to fight in himself against principles or habits characteristic of her.

For the social problem posed above, the first type of antagonism is the true parallel. And there is, at least in most cases, no obvious social harm in such a renegade-like attitude toward one's own countrymen, and in the preference for the foreigner, so long as this attitude aims only at restoration of the intra-psychic balance. In rare cases, we know, it may lead to actual treachery.

The very same intra-psychic motive may also, naturally, help the stranger in his adaptive process in foreign soil. He, too, may be more or less in the position of striving for something new and of overcoming complexes closely bound up with recollections of his past home-environment. He may similarly be moved by the sense of antagonism, or by the inner necessity for counter-regulation in response to his own family complexes. His new life, though at first only enforced by untoward circumstances, may represent for his psyche a kind of self-re-creation, a sort of rebirth. Indeed, not a few individuals whom one had to consider as social misfits full of inhibitions, or as abnormal personality-types in their native country, have derived an incentive to becoming different beings during the painful initial stage of their adaptation. The effect of the social process referred to so frequently in this work has never been illustrated through a more extensive experiment than in our times. And this on the part both of the stranger and of his environment.

3. The adaptive process of the stranger is concerned naturally with a wide range of existence. The particular colouring of thought about politics, religion, morals, and social customs; the marked differences in cooking; and, obviously, the new language, formal and colloquial, of his new country, constitute

roughly the individual fields in which adaptation first has to take place.

The present writer wishes to make a few remarks on the question of language, since he has had opportunity to view this particular aspect of the adaptive process at close quarters, and to collect his experiences from interviewing different ' strangers '. It is obvious to anybody who thinks about this topic, that speaking and conversing fulfils a double task. The first, more elementary aim, is the utilitarian [1] aspect, i.e. the seeking for information, the satisfying of one's wants, and the reaching of agreement about certain concrete questions in the course of life.

I may mention here an interesting theory propounded by Sperber, and utilized by Freud in his explanations of the sexual dream-symbols. The former author—a philologist in Upsala—thought that the first roots of a hypothetical ' primitive language ' were meant to call the sexual partner. Later, the same expressions were used during work carried out communally. These expressions, according to Sperber's conjecture, accompanied, in the form of rhythmical utterances, certain phases of the communal work of primitive man. In this way, expressions originally denoting concepts of the sexual urge and the procreative act became divorced from their original meaning, and were applied to a particular task or tool. In the opinion of Freud, this mode of speaking has been retained in the dream-symbols ; the language of dreams uses different words from the spheres of work, agriculture, etc., to express symbolically the sexual organs and the sexual act. I am unable to express an opinion on the validity of this interesting theory. Both Sperber's theory and its employment by Freud appear logical. But the theory may well fit the following part of my exposition.

The second, not less important, significance of speech and conversation—besides the above-mentioned one—is the human need for self-expression. Speech, as a means of expressing man's feelings and thoughts, i.e. his mental condition at a given moment, is, in its biological significance, comparable to the need to breathe ; it is part of human life. This second, subjective aspect of speech is, it will be admitted, clearly distinguishable from its first, utilitarian significance. If, then, Sperber's theory is right, the very first use of speech originated in an emotional source, i.e. in the need of the primitive man to call his partner. The more complicated the emotional life of man became, the more his partner meant to him, the more essential his fellow-beings were

[1] Useful and necessary.

in general for the psyche, the more extensive became the field of speech in mental life. It is clear that, in stressing this subjective aspect of speech, we are not necessarily committed to Sperber's theory.

And—to return to our original topic—the second aspect of speech is of great significance for the life of the stranger. It is difficult to employ a language so new and so incompletely under command for the sake of subjective relief of one's self. It is as if a person should always have to think before taking a breath. A new language rarely becomes so much at one with one's psyche as to be a substitute for the natural ease of one's mother-tongue. Though this is more or less the case in some people. In the experience of the author this is especially so in those for whom—as suggested above—their new environment has become an incentive and a field for a new life which they deeply desire to lead.

The acquisition of a new language is particularly illustrative of the extent and implications of the adaptive process. The foreigner, not sufficiently in command of his new language, patches up his conversation with individual words of his mother-tongue. Later, he behaves similarly when using his original, his familiar language ; he cannot avoid mixing it up with the newly acquired language. This shows that the new language has become not only part of his intellectual knowledge, but closely built into the expressive automatism of his personality. One can even dream, on occasions, in the new language, in so far as the element of speaking enters at all into the original dream-experience.

Very much depends, in the course of learning a new language, on the sentimental attitude toward the environment for the sake of which the new language is being learnt. I know, for instance, of people of Hungarian mother-tongue who spent years in the Balkans, and struggled there with a language vital to their economic existence, and yet attained far less proficiency than they had attained in English or French ; and this because they found the spiritual atmosphere or social standard of the latter countries more suitable for their individuality. These people had no knowledge of Latin, so useful for both French and English ; and therefore there was nothing, apart from the *attitudinal sentiment-factor*, that made it easier to acquire the languages of France and Great Britain during a stay in these countries, or less easy to pick up the language of their temporary domicile in the Balkans.

I am concerned here, naturally, solely with the environmental factor, to the exclusion of the no less important one : of capacity for languages, or the lack of it.[1] It is unquestionably rather cruel to condemn people for not acquiring, at an age beyond their childhood, the new language of.their new political or national environment, usually forced on them. Several highly complicate psycho-nervous factors come into operation to decide on the mastery attained. The mere desire to learn the new language, and liking for the nation speaking it, are certainly not enough. Men's energies are limited ; and an enforced adaptation takes place at the expense of spontaneity in other spheres of life. Yet the earthly life of the mortal is unique. Each day of his life is lost if filled with avoidable struggle instead of with positive life. It is one of the greatest mistakes of our organized civilization to regard many things which are only meant to be administrative conveniences as essential, and to sacrifice to them the elementary rights of man to life and happiness.

Politics, the language of the State, the religion of the State, and a certain necessary uniformization, must not be supreme aims ; they are only the framework for the refinement of individual life. To misuse such institutions, from a sense of formalism and an excessive concern for uniformity, is, in fact, one of the manifestations of disguised aggression and hatred, dealt with in Chapters IV and V. (See also Chapter XXIV (9), p. 163.)

4. In speaking of adaptation, we have generally in mind a process of a beneficial character, and one that can be approved. We must take it for granted that the individual, whilst assuming new habits, a new language, and the outlook of his new fellow-countrymen, remains untouched in his moral principles, which automatically guarantee that his reactions shall remain within legality and general morality. Naturally, if the new environment insists on a legally and morally strict behaviour, then, by virtue of expediency alone, the newcomer's moral foundation remains untouched. There is, as experience shows, no substantial risk that the fact of being uprooted from all that was felt by the individual as his stable, unshakable foundation throughout life, that this change of environment will affect the previous stability of the social character. Individual cases, freed from certain consideration of their familiar home-environment, will naturally take advantage in some respects of their new liberty. But this

[1] The existence of particular 'speech-centres' in the brain suggests obviously the factor of innate disposition for the faculty of speaking.

does not mean necessarily a fundamental change in their character. Either they have never been, deep-down, different from what they are revealed to be in their emigration ; or, and this is more important, their minor, or even major, deviations from their past stricter ways of morality and legality are not indicative of a deterioration of their basic moral structure. They retain in essential the foundations of their belief in moral principles, in justice, in humane behaviour, in fairness in business, etc.

But what should be pointed out is that there are people of a more passive, inert nature ; for them everything they were used to is a homogeneous, unitary structure. Habits of merely local significance, the language they used to speak, and, on the other hand, the basic moral principles they were taught in this language and amidst their people, all these have become one close family of ideas. And these people may find it very difficult to adapt themselves, even in externals, through a tendency to conservatism. And this conservatism itself, their attachment to the accustomed, appears to be rooted in the general stability of their human, moral foundations. They cannot break away from the formalities of their past, and adapt themselves fully to the customs and the language of their new environment ; because this would imply, for their subconsciousness, a shaking of the essential human foundations of their personality. In them the externals of life, and the essential, spiritual motives of life, have become a unity, incapable of compromise and of discriminating division. There is much in this phenomenon that is really human and worthy of appreciation. It means that their minds have spiritualized even the externals of their past life ; that the formalities have been for them more than mere containers of the essential. Unfortunately, this very conservatism may become a great obstacle to necessary adaptation and also to desirable social progress.

These facts should constitute a serious warning to those who are preparing the foundations of a new world. Do not let us view emigration too lightly ; above all, the compulsory emigration of masses. It is almost murder. That is the only appropriate name for it. It was said a few years ago that any Government has the right to do whatever it likes with its citizens ; to torture them or to expel them—it is an internal affair of the State, and there is no international obligation to interfere. If this was an opinion based on material weakness and on smallness of spiritual courage —then it was one of those inevitable illnesses of our times, directly following from the fragile constitution, and tender health, of our international organism. It was an illness following from the poor conditions in the 'preventive hygiene' of politics and international affairs. But if this opinion, voiced even from high 'democratic' places, was really a political conviction, and meant to be a well-considered programme, then one can view this sad phenomenon of our times only as a reappearance of ancient savage conditions, as *atavism* which has been proclaimed to be a 'normal' phase in history. In brief, it was a mental disease, which, according to modern analytical psychology, brings to the fore many infantile, and even more primitive, i.e. savage, mental mechanisms. The psychotic, as we know, similarly views his ideas as the only valid ones, fit for reality. And, so the present author thinks, the psychotic is more or less right; because it is the *prehistoric savage* in him who imparts to him his bizarre ideas. And in those prehistoric times beliefs of a similarly absurd character were also generally agreed upon.

CHAPTER XXI

RELIGION AND CHURCHES

1. THERE is perhaps nothing in the mental life of man comparable in quality and depth with the 'religious experience'. The belief of standing in close, personal relationship to God, to the creator and maintainer of everything existing; and the performance of certain symbolic rituals, accompanied by the similar belief that man is capable of carrying out such metaphysically important—and therefore, for the universe highly relevant—actions; and to have the certainty of being the bearer of an immortal soul,—truly, all those who confess to have no understanding, and no desire for this experience, miss something that the believers do have. Yet the experienced psycho-analyst knows well that many an 'atheist' does possess a religious belief, or such a craving for a supernatural experience and for an absolute, ethical ideology; though both in a somewhat disguised form and subconscious quality respectively.

But as to the revealed, extra-human source of religion the scientifically and psychologically trained individual is at a loss. He may even himself desire, and share, the religious belief of his fellowmen. But he cannot help admitting that there has never been, and never can be, any evidence for the divine, extra-human genesis of religion. If past generations still strongly believed and hoped that in time man might receive, or acquire, clear proofs of his general or particular belief in God, this hope vanishes more and more with every passing generation.

It is not as if we applied the same non-committal attitude to the existence of super-natural (metaphysical) or 'spiritual' phenomena in general. To do so is perhaps even narrow-minded or biased. Especially today, in the age of wireless and the artificial disruption of the atom, the merely temporary validity of any past conception of what is possible has become clear. You sit quietly in your room; there is nothing and nobody in your surroundings showing signs of 'process'[1] and life. And then you switch on your wireless-set to a given wave-length, and an abundance of voices spreads over your room. All these waves have surrounded you, have filled the space around you, and its infinite extension, even before you switched on; yet a special receiver was needed to make them perceptible to your physical senses. There are possibly with us, around us, other kinds of 'existences' too; it is hardly fair to deny this possibility on scientific grounds.

However, all this has intrinsically not much to do with the idea and the claims of religion; with the idea of 'revelation' and the extra-human origin of ethics. Yet only a very biased materialist can deny—deny with fanaticism—the eternal continuance of religious desires in man; and deny the spiritualizing effect of the cultivating in oneself of such ideologies, and of submitting oneself to such experiences. The extent of social progress, and of individual refinement, which has always been due to religion, cannot be underrated by any unprejudiced person.

2. There is, however, a peculiar thing about religious conviction which is implicitly part and parcel of it. Religion, as it were, has to be intolerant. It is based on the assumption that it stands for principles and definite kinds of ritual, which are 'godly', holy, and therefore inviolable. No human being is, accordingly, entitled to feel indulgent against those who disregard them. One may have a strong scientific conviction, or a special taste in art, and may firmly believe it to be the only right one, and yet, though defended with enthusiasm, and at times even with intolerance, no one can logically state that he stands for principles the violation of which by others deserves punishment and even extermination.

[1] This means any kind of happening.

But religious conviction is, in fact, *implicitly*, closely linked up with such a formula of exclusive validity. Though the times have gone when the consistent carrying out of this formula was generally approved ; though, under so-called peace conditions, and ' European culture ', such a principle of *active intolerance* is by law excluded from existence ; though many refined and enlightened members of the clergy, even in the innermost secret recesses of their mind, definitely reject the idea of religious persecution—still, the godliness and absoluteness of religious principles philosophically do imply condemnation or even punitive retribution against those who intentionally and persistently violate it. For the religious man to feel tolerant toward a special mode of different religious conviction, or toward individuals who are socially estimable and human in their outlook, but still agnostics, and who refuse to attribute their ethics and the management of the world to God, is in fact a compromise ; is in fact inconsistent with the historical traditions of various religions. It represents an achievement of human progress, of human intelligence, and of social sense ; but it is still an intentional compromise on the part of the religious modern individual —a compromise carried out under the influence of the *social process*.

There is another way of avoiding this appearance of inconsistency. Many clergymen, and lay people alike, would prefer to believe in a religion of pure ethics, in truthfulness and a certain degree of self-restraint, especially in the spheres of sexuality. And they would like to state that these principles alone are God's commands to man ; only the violation of these principles is opposition to God ; who is, however, not keen on punishing people even for that. It is a beautiful and psychologically and socially a very beneficial conception. But it is still a modern human invention, without much foundation in the historical tradition and development of religions.

3. Another noteworthy aspect of religion is that it makes many people, and even organizations of Churches, complacent and isolationist—in the social sense. The tacit, intra-psychic formula I am referring to could be expressed in the following way : " I am pure, free from any sin condemned by religion ; I am also charitable ; I frequently attend the services. I say my prayers with devotion ; I cultivate my religious sentiment by reading ; I am an excellent human being." This attitude has no time, and

no inner urge, for social reforms. History, and life in the present, have illustrated sufficiently this phenomenon.

Non-religious people have been naturally selfish, and socially inefficient, without the factor just described. Yet a great number of religious people do in fact crave for some ' idealistic ' sentiments which should permeate their social life ; but at the same time they do not spontaneously possess social sense enough to see the insufficient, well-nigh anti-social character of their religious complacency. The very same people, if not given a tacit sanction to their egocentric, merely self-satisfying cultivation of their higher tendencies, could be—and are in fact nowadays partly—won to a more progressive and more social kind of ethics. People have begun to realize that it is not simply God's will that millions should starve and wait patiently for the charity of their fellow-men ; that the access to worldly goods is the right of every human being ; and that a better distribution of the means of life and pleasure—and of burdens—requires, in fact, only an intellectual standard in social ethics and the conception of every man's essential significance.

You will find in the old Jewish-Christian literature, biblical and post-biblical, many ideas which conform with the modern conceptions of Socialism, or with related ideas on the rights of man. Yet it is equally true that the advocates of these ideologies had first, more or less, to break away from the contemporary religious passivity and traditionalism in order to develop these points of view fully and with more realism and to advocate them more outspokenly. And it is equally the fact that much mundane progress, both scientific and civilizatory, was first needed to arrive at that condition of mind where we are now. No previous century can show a more extensive and intensive realistic broad-mindedness of conception than ours. Unfortunately, not so in actual deeds. According to all that has been indicated above, there is a definite social-human interest in supporting religious ideology and the Churches ; in our period of history at least. But on the other hand, the realistic principles of genuine science and of more progressive individualistic conceptions on morals must not be suppressed. It is the duty of the State to protect the individual from any mental pressure ; whether it comes from idealistic religious sources or from merely selfish, exploiting, aggressive tendencies. Let us create such conditions that to be a member of a religious body would never imply superiority of power, whether social, industrial, or political. Let us have such conditions that the fact of being religious or of being a clergyman does not entail more than having chosen a special kind of ideology and ethics ; and being devoted to this specially coloured way of looking upon the metaphysical aspects of life. It is an undeniable fact that phenomena of mass psychology are very easily brought into operation by religious motives. And the employment of these mass-psychological forces for ends not quite in accordance with general social well-being has followed with natural automatism on innumerable occasions throughout human history. This perennial experience calls therefore in a modern society for particular consideration ; and, doubtless, the intelligent leaders of the Churches will themselves appreciate the necessity of such preventive State-control for the sake of true humanity and social ethics.

4. Psycho-analyses, if carried out carefully and without atheistic bias, prove beyond doubt that the majority of men of our era, deep down, do crave for some kind, and some degree, of metaphysical belief. Yet the same analyses, without exception, show also the strong doubt and opposition to the religious ideologies cherished and presented by denominations throughout the ages. This double attitude of the deeper subconscious layers results in what we call religious or moral conflict. And when psycho-analysis was only a newly invented method, and its experiences were scarce, many a too-enthusiastic analyst tried to convert his patients to a materialistic and hedonistic [1] view, and initiated new conflicts in them.

Let me summarize : There is no kind of objective evidence for any religious conception, apart from a ramification of immemorial traditions with their continuous modifications.[2] Yet

[1] Hedonistic: pleasure-seeking ; or considering sensuous pleasure the aim of life.

[2] Disguises of the religious quest are numerous. Teetotalism and vegetarianism, if carried out with obvious enthusiasm, and advocated even with fanaticism, clearly betray the operation of a factor besides the sensible interest in one's own health and in the welfare of others. I know of an exceptionally learned agnostic, the son of a high prelate, who once strongly stood out against his wife and child, when almost fainting during a journey in a warm continental country on a very hot summer day, availing themselves of a glass of beer, the only beverage obtainable at the moment. The blind prepossession in favour of Utopian world reforms, social or ethical, and not less the fanaticism of some psychological circles in attacking the heretics of their system, are doubtlessly not only substitutes for religious belief, but even indicative of a thirst for religious dogma. The latter phenomenon is unique in the history of modern science ; and it clearly coincides with the spiritual trend of our generation : the realization of the deficiencies of sheer materialism, and at the same time the difficulty of any return to religion. Many a man, whilst in logical and learned writings advocating a more adult and less petty, 'less infantile human society', easily forgets this aim when displaying his own reactions toward various concrete problems of individual and scientific life.

nothing appears farther from truth than the statement that man's metaphysical inclinations are only the result of education and terror. You can naturally suppress your metaphysical cravings ; but not without transforming them into something else ; be it into a neurosis or into a more useful self-deception. You can make it even dormant and inhibit its development. But the proof, the unequivocal proof, of the purely external, educational origin of religious sentiment in most individuals has not yet been given.

Let me finish the first half of this chapter with a very simple remark, neither scientifically deep nor otherwise very shrewd. If anyone very much devoted to his own religion, and very keen to see organized society based on the very same principle, is facing a particular step which concerns his fellowman, let him consider the following : That which occurs in mundane spheres, the joy or pain which one gives to one's fellowman—all this is certain reality ; and this consideration is essentially consistent with the denominational teachings of what the religious duty of man to man is. But all the other, more metaphysical, principles and doctrines, about the right conception of God, of sin and reward, of incidental rituals of service—all these details are controversial ; though very real to the particular believer. Do not let yourself do injustice to anybody, solely influenced by the bias of such subjective principles of belief. Consider that perhaps you may be not quite right in doing so—that you may very easily, without justification, be, as it were, the murderer of your fellow-being, of his happiness, of his elementary interests, and even of the integrity of his physical and mental health. Do not desire to take over too fully, and too forcefully, the care of his soul ; do not be unduly concerned about what might occur to him after his death. Your well-meant attempts at his spiritual salvation may involve aggression and interference with his brief mundane happiness.

5. Religious tolerance has been an important watchword of social improvement since the great French Revolution. It referred to the natural intolerance of the ardent members of the different creeds. I have mentioned above this aspect of a religious belief. I have referred to the psychological implication of an alleged possession of the 'only truth about the highest spheres of human spiritual life' ; it results in more or less accentuated animosity against those of another belief. We have explained

this intolerance by the believer identifying himself with ' the case of God ', whose claims are deemed absolute and uncompromising. However, it would mean a gross self-deception on all sides not to perceive the factor of personal insistence and the biased attachment to one's beliefs and opinions in all kinds of fights for the ' truth '. The individual, and even more whole groups, fight for a certain principle, not only because it is lofty and humane, i.e. because it is ' true ', but because it is *their principle, their truth, and their liking*. Little as ' conviction and ardent belief ' in itself can constitute the touchstone of actual truth, it is yet inevitable that the destiny of truth and justice is represented and guarded only by the strength of personal human conviction. And personal adherence and personal insistence, in respect of any principle of importance, constitutes, in fact, the only source of support and of materialization for any ' Truth '. Yet this fact, unfortunately, does not exclude that other psychological fact, that personal liking, vanity, and prestige, play a great part in any fight for or against principles.

Thus we must understand that amongst the ' agnostics ', ' freethinkers ', and materialists of different shades, too, the number of biased and aggressive fighters has been similarly substantial. It is not solely the truth, but the personal mental ' complex '—to use this psycho-analytical term—that supplies the zeal they display in attacking those of their fellowmen who differ from themselves.

Social progress does not necessarily vindicate the overpowering of a minority which is fairly happy in its traditional belief. And neither does true social improvement mean the misuse of a privileged social position, such as is enjoyed by scientists, to attack what is, after all, a source of human satisfaction, simply because this source is not modern science, but a traditional religion of any kind. Here comes in the question of what is to be considered the guiding principle of private and social life. If we insist that this supreme principle ought to be the ' truth ', then both the zealous religionists and the sometimes no less zealous representatives of the natural sciences are equally justified in their mutual intolerance. But if life and social order means human happiness and harmony—then there is a due place for the truth, i.e. the seeking after truth ; and there is also an eminent place for the principle of moderation and toleration displayed even against the dictates of one's own belief. The infallible test of value of any principle is the degree of general human harmony, and peace for body and mind, following from its application.

There are a great number of people who have no innate sense at all for religion ; though perhaps they subscribe to a lofty idea of God. Others have a desire for certain denominational rites, without, however, wishing to be 'orthodox'. No small number of believers, however, want to be logically consistent ; and they adhere to a whole system of religious belief. And all these groups are existing social strata, representing genuine human tendencies. The present writer cannot see any reason why people should not have the full support of State and international organizations for their religious life, provided they do not aspire to world-domination ; or do not aim at a privileged status by utilizing resources—economic and intellectual—far in excess of what is due to their group. The present writer wishes, therefore, to point out the 'unsocial character' of intolerance, even if it comes from scientific sources. And any decision concerning public matters, but affecting closely and deeply such peculiar spheres as traditional creeds and beliefs, ought to receive as much official consideration as is due to the dignity and happiness of people. The following must not be forgotten : The opinions of the physicist, the medical man, the psychologist, the economist, sociologist, etc., are not the exclusive outcome of their science proper ; all these distinguished people, like others, have their highly subjective likes and dislikes. And not all that they say on matters beyond the scope of their scientific domain is the product of their scientifically trained mind ; still less a direct conclusion from empirical results of research.

6. There exists also a repression of religious tendencies.[1] This fact, to which Stekel first drew the attention of psycho-analysis—and which could have been proved in numerous cases beyond possibility of doubt, can have its subsequent outcomes, neurotic or intellectual. Such, for instance, is the furious hatred against religion, displayed by some scientists, in response to their personal 'traumatic' experiences in their youth in connexion with religious education ; or in response to an inefficient repression of their religious tendencies manifestly present at an earlier age. This zeal in attacking religion and its adherents can be as blind and as passionate as was the aggressive zeal of mediaeval ages in persecuting the members of different creeds. And, it may perhaps be said, this very passion betrays its origin from sentimental attitudes, at times even its origin from repressed religious fervour.

[1] Cf. Ch. X.

No doubt empiric natural science cannot find a proper place for different assumptions of religion, apart from the idea of a 'creative Power'; and still less for different contradictory theses of religious creeds (as, for instance, the free will of man and God's foreknowledge of the future; a difficult problem for theologians of all times). But this does not invalidate the subjective, 'experiential' significance of religion for millions. The great atheistic experiment of the U.S.S.R. has been interrupted by the present war. We do not know which form of secondary psychic products would have been created by this forcible suppression and repression (the first refers to the external pressure, the second to the subsequent intra-mental process). The immediate readiness of masses in Russia openly to express their religious feelings once the beloved fatherland was in mortal danger is worthy of attention. For the modern, democratic-socialistic way of progress any forcible suppression of religious life is surely out of the question. Science and modernism have failed, so far, to present any adequate substitute to mankind. And people will continue to believe; though probably with less exclusive and less absolute belief than in the past. And this may be beneficial for general tolerance within society.

7. I wish now to make a brief survey of the relationship between the religious influence on the individual and his fitness to be a citizen of a modern society. Doubtless the 'fear of God', and the attribution of one's human behaviour to the command of a divine power, may be a firmer basis of social conduct than individual volition. And compliance with the claims of a religious community certainly trains the personality in the direction of obedience and self-restraint. On the other hand, submission to organized religious guidance decreases the intellectual independence of the individual, and makes him an easy subject of biased propaganda. He may easily be persuaded to put his particular religion, or the politics of his Church, before the general welfare, since the subconscious 'neurotic' sense of guilt present in the great majority of people feels *more* satisfied by the adherence to metaphysical postulates than to rational claims of social ethics. Any deep belief in metaphysical dogmas interferes with the freedom of mind in all spheres, whether scientific research, the forming of political opinion, or participation in social and cultural progress. It is not the particular quality of the dogma that chiefly matters; though this also may be the

case. But the fact of being tied up by an unshakable belief in and obedience to a circle of traditional ideas is naturally a ' complex ', limiting the dynamic of the mind. Such adherence may naturally greatly improve the individual's actual moral purity, and guarantee his aversion from sin and crime. But, as has been said, and as is well known, it is a certain impediment to free thinking, searching—and, in fact, at times a passive helper of reactionary social tendencies. The fewer metaphysical dogmas the religious ideology of an individual contains, the more easily the socially beneficial aspects of his being religious can go halfway to meet tendencies of human progress based on science. However, society has to be grateful for the existence of a great number of citizens who are, at least in the passive sense, moral and harmless.

CHAPTER XXII

INNER FREEDOM AND SPONTANEITY

1. ' INNER freedom ' and independence of thinking, as little as possible influenced by the forceful suggestion of ' public opinion ', is an ideal strongly advocated by different writers on sociology and psychology. It is true that a successful development of the ' self ', resulting in such inner freedom, can be considered as the climax of human standards. However, the great emphasis or rather the great hopes placed by writers on this factor are not quite justified. No doubt, if such inner freedom and independence were attainable, even for a substantial minority of people, we ought certainly to strive for it, advocate it, and further its development in the individual by every means and at any cost. The risk of the individual being subject to stupid, inhumane, biased party propaganda, and the possibility of organizing millions for aims contrary to man's true interests, would be diminished.

Yet such a state of inner independence, harmoniously combined with practical common sense and justice and tolerance, and also with all kinds of wisdom, has been and will remain no less an exception than is wisdom itself, or perfect beauty, or at least as rare as is perfect health. What we can and should aim at, is social improvement ; and this implies an improvement of individual happiness, an increase of ease in life, and a decrease of avoidable sufferings and burdens. It is certainly more promising to utilize means of organization of the State power as guiding authority, and a certain pressure of public opinion for inducing people and their communal leaders to assume a socially beneficial attitude. And this cannot be materialized on any large scale except by considering human suggestibility and readiness to submit to guidance as potent and utilizable social factors. No education toward ' independence of the mind ' can be relied upon as a preventative means and an efficient weapon against philosophies of aggression, intolerance, racial and denominational ' superiority delusions '.[1] Men will remain essentially what they have always been : humanly weak, but capable of intellectual and moral achievements, *if* guided and compelled. But this latter will always remain the task of an external superior factor, of an organized legal *State-authority*, in combination with a suitable ' *public opinion* '.

There is no doubt that environmental influences, education, and the innate foundation of the individual's mental make-up, together decide what is felt to be desirable by a person. It has been recognized by sociological writers that different social qualities such as thriftiness or enterprise, or the urge to competitive work, are more or less products of existing social and economic systems. The individual is genuinely desirous of what is fairly advantageous and safe for him, in the particular cultural and communal organization in which he happens to live. And there is, similarly, no doubt that our age, in possession of so much new and enlightened knowledge on social factors, aims and ideals, could influence the individual to pursue with subjectively genuine ' spontaneity ' such aims as are in agreement with the highest ideals—and at the same time with the concrete possibilities and necessities of our age.

2. That natural spontaneity of feeling and behaving which we admire in the child cannot be retained in the adult. The absolute necessity of educational measures in different fields of human life ; the multifarious spheres in which repression and counter-regulation of tendencies and activities have to be developed through training in youth, and maintained all through life (as explained in Chapters VI, X) ; the *social process*, i.e. the continuous influence of the environment on the individual and the necessity to be always aware of our fellowmen and of their needs ; the necessity to be aware of economic factors, of the real possi-

[1] See, however, Ch. XXIV (6), p. 143.

bilities which are open to an adult of a certain age, of a certain occupation, of a certain status (e.g. whether married or not, whether having children or not)—all these factors no longer permit the mental spontaneity that is so refreshingly peculiar to the child.

We have also to consider that the human individual, if left entirely alone, would hardly develop into a fairly harmonious personality. If not guided, educated, and trained—in short, if not influenced by the social, environmental process in a more or less regulated manner, as is done by law, convention, and the existing civilized standards—if left alone to his own automatism in his development, he would still *not* be happily spontaneous. Since the multitude of inevitable environmental influences, physical and personal, would still surround him, these influences without his reactive participation would lead to an irregular, disproportionate development of his personality. For instance, he would develop a sense of resentment against people and against the forces of Nature, owing to various restrictions and attacks on his desires and his individuality in general ; yet he would *not* develop an understanding of the causes of these phenomena, and he would not develop a sense of solidarity, would not develop the faculty of identification ; and would not even be able to enjoy the regularity of a social order maintained by others. Finally, he would become a creature distorted in outlook, and feeling himself strange in the world of others ; and he would have either to withdraw into solitude or perish in a hopeless fight for his 'natural automatism'.

The social human being develops best if guided; if aided to develop within a framework of a planned human pattern which is based on historical experience and on scientific research. In so far as the manifestation of his inclinations, the operation of his instincts, his thinking, feeling, and acting, *are trained*, he may be enabled to live in a certain mental harmony. And this harmony may give him the feeling of satisfaction and naturalness which may result in a certain degree of spontaneity. This means that the adult, if well trained in the art of life, if his mental and physical orchestra works harmoniously, may feel a satisfaction in life, may enjoy a kind of ease and spontaneity ; whilst the child's spontaneity is a natural spontaneity, due to a *lack* of experience and of adaptive development. The child is probably more cheerful (though not carefree [1]) owing to its natural spontaneity than is the adult. But the latter, if fairly harmonious, feels certainly a more intense

[1] Cf. Ch. VI.

happiness, a more extensive intellectual and emotional satisfaction.

If a person's mind is harmonious—if there is a fortunate co-operation between natural inclinations and response to external necessities, and if not exploited by the stronger, and if not forced into a group of socially or culturally under-developed masses—then the individual *is independent* ; he is able to feel and think and act in a fair independence.

3. The individual's independent active contribution toward improvement of his own emotional condition is almost negligible. It is the environment that offers, permits, or denies different desirable conditions. Within the psycho-analytical situation, too, it is the analyst—a human fellow-being, the object of the transference emotion, the interpreter of subjective puzzles, expositor of the apparent nonsense of symptoms, adviser and encourager—who does the essential work leading to emotional relief and symptomatic improvement.[1] And if we consider the various conditions that determine the integrity of the emotional self-experience (cf. Chapter VIII), then the above statement appears self-evident. Phrases such as " cheer up ", " pull yourself together ", and similar well-meant pieces of advice, have an appropriate effect for a few moments only, or so long as the available energy of the individual is capable of assuming, for the sake of social approval, a conventional smile and pose. *But essentially, only the constant environment can create, in a sufficient extent and depth, conditions under which the individual in possession of an average integrity of his mental functions can build up, or restore, the balance of his emotional-self. . . .*

And such is also the case with the moral-social aspect of a person. Just to receive encouragement to be strong, and good, and dutiful, and a patriot, and kind to everybody, is not sufficient in many cases ; since the great majority of people live under unnecessary stress, under too much dependence, under continuous threat concerning their future, and the future of their wives and children. A society which simply commands men to behave ' normally ', but shuts its eyes to the grave deficiencies of environmental conditions, private and communal, does just the same as the learned doctor who, after carefully examining his patient, kindly tells her : " You have to take care of yourself, Mrs. X ; do not worry, enjoy more rest and fresh air and sunshine, and

[1] Cf. Ch. XXIII.

everything will turn out well " ; and then he opens the door to the miserable creature and sends her back to her wretched little unhygienic house, in a smoky industrial district, to her daily life which consists in toiling for a few shillings all day, and then in the evenings receiving the ' company ' of a quarrelsome, drunken husband. But whilst the doctor, at times at least, feels deeply embarrassed after having behaved in such a hypocritical way, the law and the State are impersonal and objective, as if saying : " Do, poor creature, what you can for yourself, and keep in mind what the State doctor says : Do not forget to maintain my traditional public order."

CHAPTER XXIII

WHAT CAN THE PSYCHO-ANALYTICAL PROCESS INDICATE ABOUT SOCIAL LIFE?

1. Whilst carrying out psycho-analyses—for the past fifteen years or so—and observing the depth and the extent of what is going on in the mind of the individuals analysed—whether patients or colleagues in training—and also clearly having in mind my own training analysis and its subsequent effects, which extend practically over one's whole life, it has always been my impression that we may learn very much from this particular method for the broader field of social organization.

It has now been long recognized that the main specific feature of the analytical situation is the peculiar state of symbiosis (co-existence) between analyst and analysed person. The reader may not at first fully grasp the significance of this description. In the mind of the general public, psycho-analysis is essentially an intellectual process, consisting in enlightenment given by the analyst, who interprets, and helps to bring to the surface, subconscious knowledge in the possession of the analysed person. In fact, that which is called, in the language of psycho-analysis, the transference situation is at least as important a factor in this treatment as is the intellectual one.

Transference means that the analysand (analysed person) transfers to the analyst his dormant sentiments, the emotional attitudes (such as love, hatred, resentment, and criticism, appreciation and identification, etc.) which he originally had toward other persons who were or are significant in his life. The analysand, as it were, revives in himself, and repeats with the analyst, relationships he experienced in his past with parents and brothers and sisters, and also with particular persons who played an emotional role in his early life. Apart from this transference (which, as is easy to understand, is constantly changing in its quality in the course of the analysis [1]), there exists between the two actors of the analytical drama a relationship unique in its character. The analysand is allowed, and even encouraged by the analyst, to speak out frankly anything that crops up in his mind, to give vent to any sentiment, to express any idea, whether critical or appreciative, about anybody, himself, and the analyst included. Truly, an exceptional situation! And, it might be thought, a very pleasant situation—but, in fact, not entirely so.

Most people suffer too much from having to repress their emotional experiences and true opinions about things. They suffer from this necessity quite *consciously*. It is surely a sort of pleasure to be able to express oneself without restraint to somebody who appears to have as much understanding of human life as it is possible to have. The analyst must not be an indignant moral judge of his patient ; and if he is himself sufficiently analysed and a little experienced in life, he never does feel the moral indignation that all other people so readily feel on different occasions.

Now, it is interesting to see that the analysand takes only a limited advantage of the opportunity given to him. Sooner or later he feels that his recollections and thoughts are blocked and that nothing further comes into his mind ; he experiences what is called the *inner resistance*. And it is not only a subconscious, involuntary resistance that stops the patient's flow of speech. Many patients will tell you that they consciously do not feel like expressing certain ideas ; though on the face of it the particular idea in question, which in the end does get expressed, appears no more embarrassing than many other ideas already expressed on previous occasions, and with more frankness and readiness. The resistance in itself is a 'transferred' attitude from the past ; the analysand feels like keeping back some details which—so he thinks—the analyst would like to know. *The natural tendency toward privacy and independence which exists in man's psyche besides his desire for free expression and mutual exchange of ideas comes clearly to the fore during certain stages of analysis.* It is, as we know, already present in the child in its attitude toward the parents and teachers.

[1] Different 'transferences' being alternatively brought into operation by the subconscious, as different recollections are revived.

Privacy of life, both mental and physical, is an elementary need of civilized man. Some possess more of it, some less ; but essentially it is a psycho-biological need in us which wants to be satisfied and which creates resentfulness if disregarded. The purely social, purely communal type of man, always exhibiting himself and submitting, is not the ideal civilized man. His condition is not that in which man is in a position to develop fully to a higher ' spontaneous ' human being. No doubt, besides all the necessary sense for community and mutual regard, the desire for privacy of life has to remain the ideal condition to be made possible by society.

2. Something similar to the above-mentioned transference in analysis may occur, to a substantial degree, in ordinary social life. There are individuals enough who have a great tendency to enter very quickly into an ' emotional relationship ' with their fellowmen; the chief obstacle being, naturally, that this relationship exists mostly only in *their own volition*, whilst the other may feel no closeness toward his fellowman who ' emotionally transfers ' to him, apart from a fair amount of collaborative sentiment, as required during any common work. It may be that this second individual is emotionally satisfied through his own family life and a few good friends, congenial to his own personal make-up ; he is, therefore, not even capable of accepting the emotional friendship of the former, of his ' craving ' fellow-being. Or it may be that this second individual is emotionally shut up, for different reasons, e.g. from a tendency of self-protection against any closer friendship, or from a coldness of disposition in general.

It is easy to see how difficult social collaboration must become for an individual who readily transfers his sentimental attitudes to his fellow-worker. The true nature of the phenomenon being not consciously realized, much disappointment, silent resentment, the feeling of being disregarded, not acknowledged as equal, etc., may emerge in his psyche, and make his interest in that particular work or that particular environment slacken, and his productive energy and efficiency decrease.

That means that no individual is capable of maintaining a fair mental balance, as is desirable for a friendly, but objective, collaboration on the field of work, if not sufficiently satisfied in his private life. This may be a very significant factor both for the particular individual and for his employer, be it a private firm or the State.

In general, people are expected to be more or less uniform in their attitude to their duty. Though a tactful and clever manager of a factory may readily realize certain individual peculiarities, and may pay a personal, sympathetic attention to such a co-worker ; yet on the whole, organized mass-life does not allow for much understanding for the individual's private conditions. Work, endurance, a composed overt behaviour, readiness to tolerate moods or fun from fellow-workers, is equally required from everybody who is a member of a working (team) community. How many minor and major breakdowns—both nervous and physical—are due to such uniform conditions has been indicated in Chapter XII. The social importance of these intricate facts is obvious. And again the social psychologist feels entitled to call for more State-aided furtherance of mental health and private happiness, as suggested in different places of this work.

3. As mentioned above, psycho-analytical procedure is not quite pleasant in all its phases. It requires at times painful frankness, the exposition of the innermost recesses of the mind, open discussion of what the individual is proud of and of what he is deeply ashamed of. He has to submit, and does submit more or less readily, to the frank, objective criticism of the analyst, when the latter sums up his conclusions ; or when the analyst, as is constantly necessary, fights the inner resistance of his patient to go on with his ' confessions '. Not too frequently we have to point out to our patient that he is insincere, self-deceiving and even deceiving, that he is enjoying implicit advantages of his neurosis —and so on. And yet it is remarkable how attached the analysand remains, in most cases at least, to his analyst. There are moments of resentment, of furious ' counter-attacks '—even wishes may emerge in the dreams of the patient that the analyst should die ; but, essentially, the relationship is very deep and good. And this in spite of the fact that the analysand well knows that the analyst does *not* reciprocate ' in kind ' the emotional attachment, apart from being interested in the progress and well-being of his patient.

This fact illustrates and teaches a very important point : The human being is ready to submit to guidance, when this occurs within a free inter-human relationship. I do not refer to the submitting to medical treatment under the pressure of very unpleasant complaints, whether physical or psychical. Such an extraordinary condition makes people tolerate various measures and restrictions, though markedly painful and even objectionable. But during the psycho-analysis, even after the subjective complaints have more or less disappeared, the inter-human relationship may be maintained in an unchanged degree. And it is to this aspect that I am referring when drawing my conclusions as to the social character of man.

All that people need as a prerequisite and 'recompensation' of their submission and collaboration is more freedom of their emotional spontaneity, as usually given under our conditions of studied formalism. Naturally, people cannot experience free emotional spontaneity if they are not sure of full understanding; this, under the existing, unavoidable cultural conditions, is really not given except during psycho-analysis. Relatives, friends, fellow-workers and employers alike keep up the *double standard of emotional life*. Within their own mind they more or less consciously carry tendencies, peculiarities, cherish wishful fantasies of which the spontaneous expression, or even admission, is against social-ethical convention. And in their inter-human relationships and social behaviour they all act as if such inner experiences did *not* exist at all in them and in all 'normal' people. So much so, that a great many of our patients really believe that only *they* have hatred, accentuated sexuality, and, occasionally, so-called perverse fantasies—they are convinced that the great majority of people, and especially 'respectable people', are void of such tendencies.

Within a psycho-analysis that is proceeding well, this double-standard relationship does not exist; and, consequently, the conditions of a freer inter-human relationship are better founded. I do not want to assert that the deep emotional anaesthesia provided by the emotional transference factor may be equalled by frankness in ordinary social life. Yet careful analysis of the analytic situation, in its different phases and in different persons, proves clearly the independent existence and effectiveness of this frankness-factor; and consequently the validity of our conclusion.

There ought to be, and indeed could be, more social frankness and less of that double standard mentioned above. And this increased openness is, I think, possible without endangering the necessary degree of good behaviour and of that self-restrictive decency of feeling about things which are more or less *the most private domain of man*. These private spheres of human feeling ought to remain private, i.e. not be exhibited in their manifestations ; but their existence and their universality should be a matter of general frank agreement. And this would relieve many a man's fear of being ' discovered ' and found ' abnormal ', or less decent than those non-existent ' normals ' are in the general imagination.

And psycho-analysis proves also that even people with a deficiently developed sense for adaptation are, in most cases, only ' inhibited ' ; with better consideration for their individuality, or an improvement of their private life, they would be able to take *more part in the life and work of the community.*

CHAPTER XXIV

EDUCATIONAL FIELDS OF REFORM

1. THERE are, it has been remarked, two possible ways of planning and of constructing the foundations of a future society. The one views the progressive stage of development immediately ahead, following directly from the experience of the past. It is the way of direct progression in the concrete spheres of life, utilizing what has been plainly revealed by the deficiencies of the past and present. It works through giving up some attempts and established institutions of the immediate past ; whilst correcting, enlarging, and supplementing others. The Beveridge plan,[1] for instance, is essentially such a design. It is fundamentally based on a social principle more or less operative in our present structure of State-organization. The duty of the State to care for certain minimal requirements of all its citizens in exchange for the organized behaviour of the individual is a principle already recognized, though only very inadequately materialized up to now.

No doubt such general improvement of the average standard of living should have its beneficial psychological consequences. Better housing, less worry about the basic necessities of life, should implicitly improve, to a certain degree at least, the inner atmosphere of the family ; it may decrease mental tension and leave more amplitude for the freedom of the mind, more ground for a satisfactory emotional experiencing, a firmer basis for spontaneity

[1] Czechoslovakia had a somewhat similar, though short-lived scheme of social insurance for all people in employment, but of more limited financial scope, in accordance with the national economic potentialities.

in feeling, in thinking, and in the normal enjoyment of daily life.

Deep down in everybody's psyche there is a simple, uncomplicated, unsophisticated soul, easily satisfied by the necessary amount and necessary kind of nourishment, sunshine and air, peace and ease, and by a fairly friendly, sympathetic, and loving environment.

All those individualistic manifestations of striving, planning, fighting ; all those undesirable phenomena of envy, jealousy, cunning, and hatred ; all those tendencies aiming at power, at dominating, at being ' above ', constitute, in the opinion of the author, *a second layer*, a superstructure of the human personality. Those who carry out psycho-analyses, and especially the more passive, expectant kinds, know from their experience what calming-down, easing, and buttressing-up of the personality is instituted by this procedure. This occurs chiefly through giving the patient the opportunity to enter into a free, more or less uninhibited human emotional relationship with someone who is educated, experienced, and understanding enough to grasp, explain, and forgive the deepest emotional manifestations of his fellowman. The analyst not only does not object, but even encourages his human fellow-creature to give free vent, by verbal expression, to all that he desires to experience ; and also to transfer to the analyst, alternatively or simultaneously, the various sentimental attitudes he is bearing in himself.

We may assume, therefore, that the better satisfaction of the above *elementary personality-layer* will have its beneficial effects on a man's whole behaviour as a social being. It will, to a certain degree at least, influence the spheres of those complicate tendencies described above, which I have conceived as a superstructure of the personality. But I think there is *no* justification for limiting social planning only in this direction. There is no justification for tackling only those aspects, for improving only those fields of human existence, on which the attention of the Socialist has been focused so far, and not without justification. We have, in the meantime, learnt much more about the deeper nature of human manifestations within the social community.

2. In the past there was constant criticism because the school curricula put too little emphasis on natural and ethnographical sciences and too much on classical, grammatical studies, the core of educational material in past centuries. Nowadays the teaching

of natural sciences, and also of modern languages, is better adjusted to the requirements of our concrete life. But a still more serious gap remains—the absence of education in the 'science of individual and social life'.

Is it not justifiable to claim that the State should provide facilities for every youth and adult to become acquainted with at least the necessary minimum of knowledge on sexuality, on emotional life, on marriage, on birth control, on the psychology of racial and religious hatred, on the only limited validity of current beliefs and of individual opinions, and on the substantial subjectivism of human thinking and judging in general? Why do we have scientific organizations, why are we so proud of our up-to-date standards, if we keep the accumulated knowledge exclusively for the few fortunate and research-minded people? Do we not spread the results and aspects of general hygiene among the general population? What justification is there for depriving the masses of social knowledge and the knowledge of social hygiene, and not placing before them—compulsorily if need be [1]—those established facts of which the knowledge could certainly save so many bitter hours of remorse, and preserve so much working energy and so much human happiness?

It is probable that if millions of sensitive individuals were made freer of neurotic conflicts during their early youth, during the important years of preparatory development, the social tension in their life as adults would become less: and the general productive capacity, as well as the capacity for happiness, would be increased. First of all, the doctrine that human physiological needs are essentially filthy must be thoroughly eradicated. There is certainly another way, an improved way, of educating younger and older children toward 'decent' behaviour in daily life, toward cleanliness, and toward keeping the physiological functions, whether they relate to excretion, or menstruation, or the sexual urge, as a sphere more or less private and guarded by a moderate degree of shyness. The retention of these principles will always remain part and parcel of our culture; and they actually are natural tendencies of the developed human mind. There is no doubt that the mind of man does find a spiritual satisfaction in keeping these spheres shrouded in privacy; and it is certain that much refinement in other spheres of the mind has followed this 'repression'.

But it is equally true that there is *no need at all* for instilling the idea into the plastic young mind that these things are 'inferior'

[1] Cf. Ch. XXVI, p. 163.

and are only tolerated because they have to exist ; and that they are essentially antagonistic to the ' spirit ' and the metaphysical soul. There are a great number of people with a firmer mental constitution who, though intimidated by such educational measures in their homes and at school, finally overcome these influences ; they are able to realize that these strict principles are not to be taken literally, and they carry on with life without continual mental conflicts. But another great section of the people remain more or less lifelong captives of this solemnly imparted ideology. And in consequence they suffer constantly from more or less intense mental conflicts between what they still occasionally do and have to do, and what they believe they ought to do, in keeping with the ascetic, religious, ' unfleshly ' ideal.

We know for certain that the overwhelming majority of such fights against ' the flesh ' serve no useful, no truly spiritual purpose. They serve mainly to keep down human productive energy and to reduce inner independence; reinforcing the limitations imposed on people legally and by virtue of necessity by the State, and also the suppression carried out from individual motives arbitrarily by the stronger and more efficient people exploiting their weaker fellowmen for their own purposes. It is surely a shame for mankind, endowed with science and intellectual dignity, that mistakes are cultivated and misinterpretations taken advantage of to keep the individual in legal fetters ; that such ways and means of ' social education ' are utilized to make the human creature into a weak and easily led law-abiding citizen, tolerant in attitude, and enduring.

3. I was once asked to write a foreword to a popular work on general medical and psychological principles, which was to be published for special use by a large youth organization cultivating high ethical principles. I asked the author first to correct his statements about the great harm attributed in past ignorant centuries to the so-called erotic self-satisfaction (masturbation). This enlightening passage (copied from a book written just 120 years earlier) contained threats of subsequent tuberculosis, of brain diseases and early senility, and of every sort of earthly ill. The well-meaning author replied : " I know. I have read modern views on this topic ; but I think it is worth while to startle the imagination of youth in order to reinforce his moral sentiments." My answer was : " I realize and appreciate your

high aims ; but I certainly do not feel justified in supporting your method. I think it is cruel to deny the facts, especially to those whom we love and appreciate, and to let them suffer agonies of fear ; a fear which they are bound to experience, since there is—as you know from your own past life—no way of entirely eradicating the sexual urge in youth before marriage. Why on earth should I deny the facts, and cause terror to those idealistically minded boys whom we appreciate ; whilst others, less thoughtful and less scrupulous, may enjoy a mind at rest, and even free access to the results of sexual-psychological research ? Try other ways and means of spreading moral sentiments. Where is the morality of a principle which cannot be maintained without lying threats ? "

4. Another very important point on which general enlightenment should be given to both parents and children is the complicated relationship of the two generations. The tension between the educating adult and the educated junior is inevitable. The occasional outburst of the parent and teacher on the one hand, and on the other hand the intelligible resentment in the psyche of the child and pupil when being restricted and guided, is also not only ancient but for ever inevitable. And it should by no means be still believed by ' children ' of all ages that to experience antagonism against parents on some occasions is a deadly crime and the nadir of moral insanity. The great number of neurotic complexes based on this strong belief, and the continuous conflicts between feelings of resentment toward parents—inevitable as they are—on the one hand, and the religious conscience on the other, means a waste of energy and working efficiency. It is naturally impossible to find a clear solution for the practical aspect of the problem ; it is impossible to eradicate its painful existence and its occurrence in every family. In education there must be a certain authority and even force, and perhaps even a theoretical threat of punishment. But it is equally true that intelligent parents themselves could do much to brighten the home atmosphere and to lessen the fear and tension ; and clearly they are never justified by any logical consideration in spreading terror and belief in their ' divine superiority ' ; though the old biblical ideal does require or approve of this. However, for the individual of our era such a demand, if taken literally, has been proved intolerable. It is difficult to ' adore ', single-mindedly and unconditionally, a human being who himself is full of

imperfections, himself so unmistakably displaying personal vanity and the desire for unopposed authority, and showing to a more or less but always considerable degree his liking for the pleasures of the palate, for mundane comfort, and, last but not least, for the tabooed sexuality. And even for the smaller child, not yet in a position to realize all this—though we certainly underrate its early capacity of seeing, sensing, and understanding—one thing is pretty sure : that grown-ups find his childish likings and plays 'unbecoming, filthy, sinful', etc., because they themselves can easily dispose of all that, owing to their different interests and different sources of satisfaction.

All this, and similar knowledge, is largely a part of everyday hygiene. And the absence of such knowledge is largely a source of risk to mental health in the earlier or later years of the individual, just as the lack of elementary information on cleanliness and on the avoidance of infection entails a menace to the maintenance of physical well-being. From where shall such important knowledge be derived, if not from the educational institutions maintained by the State? Or shall we still leave all this information to the psycho-therapist, who has to treat by hard work, at the cost of much time and expense, those who have broken down, chiefly because of their unregulated way of life, left to untutored automatism ; a life for which there was an excuse only in past centuries through the utter lack of research and knowledge in this field? Here, too, prevention is better than cure. Everyone admits and fully realizes that the individual personality has considerably changed during the ages ; parallel with all the alterations in civilization and organized social life. Is it not only logical that his mental complications must be reconsidered in the light of this new way of life?

The present-day boy and girl, man and woman, cannot meet all the requirements of life with a sufficient supply of nervous energy if burdened with unnecessary conflicts, based only on mistakes. They have the right to know something of the complicated emotional processes that occur, consciously and subconsciously, in the psyche, in the course of its efforts to 'digest' the difficulties and the contradictory sentiments arising from the living together of educating parents and educated and guided children.

There are still many people who are greatly disturbed by the realization of their mixed sentiments toward their nearest relatives, and especially parents. Each of them thinks he is entirely exceptional "because he is not ethically minded and dutiful enough ". Why deny man the knowledge of the universality of such complications? Some parents would gladly do anything to diminish the conflict in the minds of their children if they only knew how! But they have long forgotten all that they themselves experienced in the past. And if they are still aware of their own critical sentiments toward their parent, they hardly apply this knowledge spontaneously to the relationship between themselves and their children; since " they are certainly different "; ' they ' meaning both the parents themselves and their children.

5. There are educational reasons for devoting careful thought to the problem of the application in education, in the light of present social conditions, of the *strictness* that was customary in the past. But there appears to be particularly imperative need for careful consideration of *education in the moral concepts* to which our civilization subscribes, but which are frequently transgressed by the adults, the educators of the children. The educative principle that lying, insincere, or evasive replies are indicative of an obscure moral character, is within the psyche of the child frequently ' counteracted ' by the impressions of lies which the parents habitually employ in their social and business life; they do so in part from ' conventional social cowardice ', but also to a substantial degree from the motive of defence of their own and their families' interests. But the shock is inevitable when the psyche of a sensitive child first realizes that this double standard of morals is operative in his mind. Through the process of identification both educational influences retain their dynamic power.

Even more disastrous is the shock—leading to grave inner conflicts—if the child has to realize that his parents are not proof against the minor attractions and temptations of sexuality. The coquettish smile of a vain young mother, directed toward a strange man, has embarrassed many a sensitive child who has been taught that *any sign* of erotic inclination is immoral, and who has been made to believe that the mutual fidelity of his parents surrounds them with an impregnable wall of indifference to members of the opposite sex. I am referring to what has been explained on this topic in Chapter IX (6), page 51. There must surely be a way of imparting sufficient moral education without overstressing to the yet immature child the absoluteness and gravity of our moral laws. The inevitable disappointments in this respect experienced by children in respect of their parents or of other adults will result in a smaller shock if the general tone of education is less emphatic and less intimidating. After all, the thorough carrying out of those moral principles is chiefly the task of the adult. And accordingly, the due seriousness of these principles should perhaps be considered and realized only by the more matured youth ; whilst the younger children should learn rather the refined and beautiful aspects of our moral principles, in preparation for a more complete appreciation of their deep significance in later life.

This is a very serious suggestion, differing greatly from our customary ideas on education. The author is fully aware of all the educational and social difficulties attached to his suggestion. But the true facts of life, of its customs and social formalities, and of its temptations, should seriously be considered when choosing an expedient path of modern education. There must be a path leading toward the acquisition of a well-developed moral sense, while at the outset, in dealing with early youth, it is surrounded more with the attractive aspects of morality than with its seriousness, at times involving tragically grave situations.

6. There is nothing more important for progress in humanity than increasing education of masses, both in particular knowledge and in the faculty of logical thinking. Far-seeing leaders and visionaries may make their prophetic summons to the ‘ social conscience ’, and may be the originators of modernized conceptions. But it is the amount of knowledge and the degree of independence of thinking on the part of millions that decide the ultimate role of progressive conceptions in actual life. It is the weighty resolve of millions to observe those standards of living that is able to guard social life against the reactionary inclinations of a few.[1] The utter reluctance of the same millions to lend their consent and collaboration to the forging afresh of their fetters, implied by social and cultural regression, becomes the fertile soil from which mankind’s freedom and happiness spring. The vision and idealism of a few leaders and creative minds cannot alone accomplish this.

The contempt for the masses, and for their ‘ gullibility ’ and intellectual passivity in various periods of history is, from the viewpoint of dynamic psychology, unjustifiable. It would be lamentable if millions of thinking people fully realized the folly

[1] It is not so much the reactionary striving of the few ‘ would-be lords ’ that is to be feared as the passive acceptance of this ideology by the masses.

and backwardness of the ideologies utilized in the maintenance of a social order beneficial only to a minority, and were still unable to live to see at least signs of a change in the course of their own generation. This would imply for them suffering almost beyond endurance. It was an age-long blessing for the masses to be able to believe that their poverty was ordained by God, and that there was true virtue in enduring social oppression and gross injustice with devout resignation ; and to consider their lowly fate only as a means of spiritual purification, sent by the divine wisdom for the actual benefit of their souls. Through this religious ideology they developed genuine virtues of undoubted value. Still more important, this process of ' social adaptation ' saved them from despair and ' panicky ' frame of mind, which certainly must have been their share if they had clearly realized the *mainly human sources of their sufferings*. It is good that, at any period, only a few specially gifted ' prophetic realists ' should know the full possibilities of social improvement ; that *they* should gradually educate the masses until the time comes when there is a possibility of achieving it. Increasing knowledge and spreading intellectual enlightenment can undoubtedly contribute toward a quickening of such a progressive social process. But unquestionably there are certain limiting laws of Nature (perhaps even metaphysical) which necessitate phases of quiet preparatory development.

This remark naturally does not imply any support for a factual limitation of education and enlightenment of the broad masses. Its purpose is only to explain the fact of the self-deception of the masses and its beneficial and regulative aspect. This phenomenon is simply another form of the well-known process called ' repression ', present in the psyche of the individual. This individual repression, too, is a beneficial and even a necessary factor. It serves to transfer to the subconscious any unpleasant and unbearable knowledge, any knowledge that exceeds the healthy capacity of the conscious mind.

The duty of the intellectual leaders is nevertheless to educate ; and to do so as much as possible. That beneficial self-blindness, enabling people to carry on amidst difficulties, will always exist to a necessary degree ; mostly, as we know, it maintains itself to excess.

7. The main difference between the traditional academic psychology and the modern type is the closer relatedness of the

latter to everyday life and its varieties and complexities. The psycho-analysis of Freud, and still more the Individual-psychology [1] of Adler, also mark a change in this respect. But an up-to-date social psychology cannot live up to its task and ideal unless it takes the objects of its research from the kaleidoscopic stage of actual social life. Science, essentially, investigates given phenomena ; and only after conclusions have been drawn from this part of research does the possibility present itself, and therefore the task, of applying some of the new knowledge for planned and constructive activity.

The present writer thinks, for instance, that the discussion of films, however briefly, should on no account be omitted from this small volume on social research and social reform. I know of hardly any other device or cultural institution of the present day that plays so important a part in the mental processes governing the masses as the cinema. People go there not simply to spend their leisure ; they obviously go there because they receive something that supplements their life of concrete reality. They go there to *satisfy their fantasy—a satisfaction which is an essential part of the life of the individual.*

It is in the main sexual problems and the large field of the struggle for bread, money, and position, that attract people's interest ; to a lesser degree they derive satisfaction from a just and happy end of a plot, vindicating the supreme validity of the educational principle : " Be good and you will be blessed." The lifelike presentation in the ' movies ' appears better fitted to satisfy the imagination of the people than books and lectures presenting in mere words the triumph of virtue and of justice.

I am perhaps not greatly mistaken in saying that the vicarious satisfaction of sexual and aggressive tendencies, providing compensation for what concrete life has not given to the individual —love, happiness, appreciation, success, position, supremacy— constitutes the main gift which the ' movies ' are able to present, with such variation and regular frequency, with such appeal to individuals of all types, on a scale which has apparently been approached by nothing else yet known in social history. The overwhelming majority of people feel more or less frustrated, feel more or less a tendency toward revenge and aggression, under the influence of the particular conditions of their life. And there is no doubt about the satisfaction-value of the cinema-plays on this point. By the process of identification with the actors of the

[1] The expression, as used by Adler, refers to the *unity* of the personality in aiming, behaving and producing neurotic character-traits.

play the spectators gain a temporary satisfaction of their own ambitions and of their tendencies to revenge.

Still more obvious is the temporary satisfaction and compensation for subjective deficiencies in that other sphere of human life, love and sex. I have used the expressions compensation and satisfaction. For these are, in fact, two different thirsts that can be quenched through the enjoyment of the 'pictures'. The first type of fantasy-compensation is that for elementary, socially justified expectations which the average individual cherishes, but the fulfilment of which frequently falls short of his hopes.

A modest and warm-hearted girl marries a similarly modest boy, who, like her, wishes to find a loving and sincere companion for life. They both dream of deep and eternal happiness, and they promise it to each other. The first years of their marriage are, however, full of the struggle for existence, and for the bringing up of their child, born in the first year. There is still, undoubtedly, much left of the love of the first months, but the fatigue of the day, and the cares of the economic struggle, force the manifestation of this love more and more into the background of mere good intentions. Soon, however, the small business develops; the husband, previously tied up by the difficulties of narrow financial means, now becomes occupied with the troubles of a big business. His commercial interests require social intercourse with other, even bigger business-men, in hotels, in clubs, and at sports meetings; whilst his wife, essentially still a modest wife, and mother now of two small children, stays mostly at home. There is no sign of infidelity on his side, or of conscious dissatisfaction; but there is little cultivation of love, still less any increase of love, only a friendly co-existence without either having time for the other. Regularly on week-ends both go out together to the 'pictures' and enjoy the love-happiness of elegantly dressed actors, enjoy the passionate meetings of imaginary people—and they are compensated for what they themselves have not, for what they cannot have, owing to ignorance at the start of their marriage, and no less owing to the social conditions of our age, which absorb the weak individual entirely into the acquisitive process of business and production.

Now an illustration of the other kind of *satisfaction*. There is a decent girl, well educated and charming, whose only admitted plan for life is to marry an educated and kind-hearted professional man. In this she succeeds. The young man, in addition, is quite handsome, though far removed from the athletic actor, and certainly not a 'lady's man'. He is greatly in love with his charming wife ; and she, too, seems to be happy. At times they go to the cinema, and more frequently to a 'show' ; and, to the surprise of the serious and strictly monogamic husband, his charming wife never stops being enthusiastic about the 'sweetness' and the 'handsome figure' of this or that actor, about his 'beautiful smile', and similar things. The embarrassed husband cannot join in the praise, since he begins to have feelings of inferiority ; above all, he is puzzled, because many of the men on the stage who are admired by his wife are, in his opinion, anything but strikingly handsome. I know this from his complaints during a training analysis : I also had the opportunity of knowing his wife more closely before she was married to him, and I am satisfied that she is a decent wife, and also that she would never have thought of marrying an actor or an opera-singer, however handsome. Her conscious aims were always directed toward science, a monogamous, happy marriage, and a religious spirit in the home ; and all this is hardly to be expected in the general run of actors.

The solution is clear : the charming wife does not even realize how polygamous she, in fact, is ; how much within her psyche she is craving for the love or attention of famous and elegant actors, who, however, are at the same time the ideal of numerous other girls. Not that our woman would in reality exchange her husband for such a one. Had she the choice once again, and the opportunity of choosing between both types, undoubtedly she would decide again for that type which her husband represents. The other man is only the object of her fantasy-life ; she, though unaware of this, wishes to enjoy him, but simply and solely during her occasional revelling in a 'picture' or a 'show'. The realm of fantasy—far from actuality—is the field of her longed-for satisfaction, desired by her 'polygamy' complex. This is consequently a satisfaction, but not a compensation for what is being wished in concrete actuality, consciously wished but not entirely attained.

People under psycho-analysis not infrequently dream about particular scenes they have seen in the 'pictures'. They naturally refuse at first to submit such a dream to analysis, stating that it is simply a reproduction. But, in fact, one can frequently find that the part of the film picked out by the dream-process has an intrinsic bearing on the deepest problems, mostly difficult conflicts, of the dreamer. A young man suffers much from jealousy because of his fiancée's behaviour, but because of his passionate attachment to her he cannot decide to break off the engagement.

He sees the picture ' Pittsburgh ', and in his dream of the following night he finds himself in a merry company at a dance. He recognizes the origin of this dream-motive from the picture of the previous night, where there were two scenes of a dance. He realizes, however, only with the help of the analyst, who happened to know the picture, what is being hinted at by this dream. One hero of the play is an energetic but not quite reliable man, who, because of financial ambitions, marries the daughter of a steel magnate, but thinks that he can keep up his intimate friendship with a girl whom he loves ; the latter, being of a good character, refuses to agree. There are two scenes of a dance at which the fiancée, and later wife, of the unscrupulous young man meets the other girl. No doubt the dream-fragment expresses the secret wish of the dreamer to be also unscrupulous enough to marry a ' decent woman of social position ' and somehow to keep up simultaneously the passionate relationship with the girl he irrationally likes but intellectually despises.

But, as has been said, visiting the cinema means to most people, on frequent occasions, at least a substantial satisfaction. And implicitly a poisonous factor. Because ' pictures ' mostly present solutions that are far from being real possibilities. The acting figures of plays are mostly unmarried, or else without children or dependent relatives to care for. They can wish, and aim at, almost anything ; and even if in the play they meet with handicaps, they do many things, and attain things, which are entirely out of reach for the average human being. ' Pictures ', whilst satisfying the psyche for two hours, operating after the fashion of alcohol or a sedative drug, may drop into the mind the additional seed of the desire for the unattainable, instead of solving the difficulty.

I have pointed out how unsuccessful marriages—and unsuccessful careers in general—are mostly the result of neurotic inhibitions and subconscious tendencies. The ' pictures ' dramatically describe the existing tragedies of life—but the only remedy they advise is : intrigue, aggression, and adultery ; and all this in a way exceeding the real possibilities for average men and women. Surely the great success of films is indicative of the fact that they do give something substantial to the public. However, they could give more : true life and true solutions, or hints at prevention. I am not thinking of the usual propaganda films, in which the artificiality of the setting and the tendency is so obvious ; nor of that type of lukewarm sentimentalism the remoteness of which from true life is manifest to everybody. I mean a more serious type of art produced with the help of the highest institutions of public education and science, supported by the State, and finally in fact appreciated by the wider public. People should learn to live ; youth should be given illustrations of why and how to avoid situations that lead inevitably to insoluble difficulties.

Above all, the 'pictures' stimulate eroticism undesirably—a process *in marked conflict with our actual social need* of self-restraint and sublimation ; and they attack the ideal of monogamous love. Though to interfere with such a state of affairs is against the principle of freedom ; yet to do so to a certain degree, for the sake of the well-being of people, for the sake of their better mental harmony, is to serve at least as important a social need as that of unlimited freedom. After all, there is no total freedom for the consumption of alcohol—scandalous behaviour of the drunkard is opposed by the authorities—and nobody invokes in this respect the principle of freedom.

In creating and supporting a really intellectual type of film production,[1] and gaining more or less public approval for the more realistic type of 'picture' as suggested above, interference with the other type of film may even prove superfluous. *The social process* itself may turn the taste and the requirements of the masses into a more desirable direction ; and the enjoyment of that other type of film may be limited to the psychopaths, or to exceptional moments in the life of 'normals'.

8. Science of all ages has been inspired by two aims—that of searching for new facts and technical devices, and that of interpreting given phenomena. The first type of science finds its corrective and regulative factor in the apparent success or failure to achieve advance.

The particular methods of modern natural sciences, and their application in life, are, therefore, fairly safe and expedient. This is not so in that other field of the creative intellect, which mainly interprets and suggests theoretical theses and principles. Philosophy and psychology, and the application of their methods to social psychology, are not only subject to marked subjectivism, but to grave mistakes.

The interpretative scientist, especially the psychologist, cannot avoid working on the foundation of his own subconsciousness and on that of his individual mental make-up as a whole. He does

[1] This does not necessarily mean restricting films to the 'serious' type.

so, in the same way as everybody does, by building for himself a *Weltanschauung* or outlook on life. The particular features of one's own nature and capabilities are bound more or less to influence such an individual system, with its implicit aim of finding a favourable place and justification and explanation for one's own personality. To employ a very simple instance :

A person with a handsome appearance is apt to stress, in his conception of the human society, the role of externals ; whilst another person, less fortunate in this respect, must prefer a system of ideas in which the bodily factor occupies less place, and mental qualities, such as decency or cleverness, enjoy the main emphasis.

Or, if an individual is well fitted for sublimating his instinctual tendencies, he will more readily subscribe to, and advocate, an ideology comprising strict sexual morals, and praise a world without aggression, and full of appreciation and reward for science, arts, religion, etc., as the case may be in respect of himself.

The obvious reluctance to acknowledge a psychology of the subconscious, peculiar to so many people, springs from similar motives. Its acceptance implies an admittance of the possible existence of disapproved motives in the individual. Nobody likes to believe in principles which may, on some point or other, imply an accusation and condemnation of his own personality. And nobody chooses easily an ideology which would imply a measure of value very critical and censorious of his own mental standards.

The one-sidedness of contemporary psychological systems comes not only from the limited horizon of every mortal, but chiefly from this subjective bias of the scientist. But this surely does not detract from the justification of individually coloured systems. There are always thousands and millions to whom a particular psychological system may apply ; and there is much in every system that *is part of the whole truth*. Naturally, by stressing one particular aspect, a distortion may follow ; and for particular cases it may imply a mistake when applied in treatment and education. At times the *extract* of a whole may leave out details which are very important and are not represented by those details which are contained in the scheme. For instance : Everybody needs guidance, help, and friendship. But whilst the mind and the emotional balance of *one* individual is not satisfied without experiencing an emotionally coloured relationship with his superior or collaborator, another person's mind may be satisfied by the simple fact of being supported and helped. To insist, *in the first case*, that the overcoming of the inferiority feeling by the fact of collaboration alone is the chief socio-psychological factor to be considered, would soon prove a mistake, if the guiding and helping person should be of the type that is unable to evoke and display the signs of emotional friendship so greatly needed and greatly missed by the person helped.

The relationship between a theory and the particular practice in the same field is frequently not very close ; but in the field of educational and psycho-therapeutic measures it is perhaps even less so. The layman is not unjustified in asking how all these divergent theories can be equally valid ; and particularly how it is, for instance, that one may get equally good therapeutic results whether one happens to be a genuine Freudian or a follower of Stekel's method, an adherent of Jung's psychology or an enthusiastic student of Adler's approach.

Much could be said to explain to the uninitiated the true facts ; and to show him that there is less contradiction about the essence of the phenomena than there appears to be in their partial presentation. I should like, however, to point out one special aspect, related to the exposition in Chapter VIII. And this is the undeniable fact that everybody's mind needs a certain theoretical foundation, a certain accumulation of theses into a system, for the benefit of the individual's own emotional stability. To employ a very gross analogy : If a person sits in the open on the ground, with his arms leaning against a tree in order to support himself, and he is engaged in blowing playfully at those lovely flowers the petals of which fly so easily into the air—no doubt there is not much *intrinsic* causal relationship between his being supported by the ground and the tree on the one hand, and the active energy displayed by his breath on the other. This is, of course, only a gross analogy, perhaps not even the best one. And similarly I suggest that the adherence to a certain system of beliefs may satisfy the psyche, may increase the fundamental productivity of the mind, yet without being the direct soil of a certain plan or activity. Though the individual scientist, by virtue of his being human, prefers to state that there *is* a close and causal connexion between the two.

The education of people in psychology seems an elementary necessity of modern life, as any reader of this work will surely agree. But it presents a serious problem. The first task of a social psychology ought to be to consider how much modern analytical psychology can be popularized without doing harm to a great number of emotionally unstable people. Psychological enlightenment not only appeals to the intellect but affects subconscious spheres. Many a man has had headaches and sleepless nights after having first read a chapter in Freud or the tragic case-stories in the publications on the subject. I cannot deny that a great number of people, educated on traditional non-analytical principles, may feel embarrassed and even perturbed by psycho-analytical literature of the Freudian type. It may stimulate their subconscious complexes, and do harm which for them outweighs the intellectual benefit. There are books, as for instance the popular educational books published by Stekel, which are free from this risk. His *Primer for Mothers* (*Briefe an eine Mutter*) has been translated into twenty-six languages.[1] There are other books, too, which are cautiously written and suitable for use for popular education. Without doubt the study of Adlerian literature is not only quite harmless, but very useful for everybody. And the present author, though himself a post-Freudian psycho-analyst, feels that it is necessary to ask writers and lecturers who wish to spread psycho-analytical conceptions to be more careful than has usually been the case. The due intra-psychic digestion of some psycho-analytical disclosures can only occur in the course of well-conducted psycho-analysis. There are, however, a number of results the knowledge of which is absolutely necessary for education and Social Psychology. The author has tried to include such points in his discussions. The over-sensitiveness of a few, almost neurotic individuals, who feel perturbed by the smallest amount of psycho-analysis, must naturally be neglected for the sake of the needs of the large majority. They would be upset *in any case* through other events in ordinary life, which is so rich in stimuli for subconscious abnormal complexes and conflicts.[2]

There is another difficulty. Scientists, as a rule, are biased in favour of their subject and of their particular theories. And psycho-analysts are, in addition, reflective personality-types, each prone to concentrate on certain intricate aspects of this broad field for speculation and theorizing. It is a particular proneness toward an abstract way of thinking and reflection that makes them turn to psychology as the field of their research. Many of them are deep thinkers, moral-philosophers, reformatory minds, and in the way of prophets, keen to spread knowledge and to win general acceptance for their conviction. But it is not always certain that the material presented by lecturers on psychology is

[1] The English edition is unfortunately not up to date.
[2] It is true, however, that some books did prove mental traumas for some youth.

really the best suited to make the student benefit, the student whose prime concern is to become a better human being, a better parent, and a better citizen. It is an old law of physiology that a stimulus has different effects according to the particular condition of the stimulated living organism. The effect on the mind of the students of a lecture on psychology is not always the effect aimed at and expected by the lecturer. As a rule, *their* intellectual and emotional background is different from that of their tutor; and his definitions and expositions, though unequivocal to himself, may be *differently apperceived* by the minds of the listeners. Apperception is not only an intellectual function. Especially concepts of psychology appeal to subconscious and emotional spheres too, and their proper understanding on the part of an individual who is *not* particularly trained in this mode of thinking is greatly 'blocked' by the various repressions, operative in the normal. The theoretical psychologist, not experienced in analytical practice, is frequently not quite able to see and overcome this difficulty in teaching.

Those of us who are concerned with public education should carefully examine themselves. The educational authorities, too, should pay a little attention to this aspect. But it would be a great pity if those who are original and progressive should be prevented, because of their originality, from giving their best to the community. Discretion should be the guiding rule here.

9. The present writer finds—though this may sound very assuming—that in the application of psychological theses to the interpretation of social facts, science has so far failed to produce many workers of an *eclectic* type. And the result of this is the insufficient attention paid by men of concrete activity in politics and administration to psychological aspects and suggestions.

Moreover, we do not yet possess a sufficient number of individual psycho-therapists who are of the type that is fitted to work on the lines of *social prevention*. In the past we neuro-psychiatrists have been trained and made to fit ourselves for the treatment of neglected cases of maladaptation with grave neuroses; and the whole profession tended more or less to concentrate on the treatment of a few, preferably financially independent, individuals. This is naturally the fault of conditions. The best psycho-therapist, even with an international reputation, is severely restricted in his earning capacity, owing to the time necessarily taken up by each case; and at the same time it is advantageous for him, for his reputation, and for therapeutic success in all his cases, to be fairly well-to-do. There is nobody who, deep down, admires prestige and financial success more than the individual who is himself inefficient in this or any other respect. He may declare that " money is nothing, humanity is everything " ; his subconscious, more primitive complexes are imbued by the true conditions of economic and social life : and this, his 'primitive layer', hates his own poverty or lack of success and despises the economic limitations of the doctor if he, the patient, happens to know about them. This is a serious problem in itself ; and at the same time illustrative of *the relationship of individual mental conditions to the social and economic structure of any period.*

CHAPTER XXV

A QUESTION TO OUR CONSCIENCE

1. We have to ask each other as simple human beings, and not without some uneasiness—and again to ask ourselves as jointly responsible members of State organizations, more loudly : " What would have happened if the present war, with its disintegrating effect, had not given a jolt to the slow and torpid course of social history, had not impressed upon us a sense of the urgency of reforms, of the need for reviewing past conceptions, for considering a more or less substantial surrender of our privileges —each in his sphere of effort and of the utilizing of others for his own benefit ? If the belief in the ' eternal ' continuity of the ' existing ' had not been interrupted, how and when would any improvement have started ? "

Provided we had all our present social institutions ; an unlimited capitalism and individual enterprise, a free Parliament with new elections as frequent as desired ; and also the customary ethical propaganda of Churches and other organizations with kindred aims ; and also the greatest number of periodicals, books, and lectures appealing to the ' better part ' in man, to his intellect, to his soul, to his sense of justice ; and provided also that, by efficiency of all this public instruction—or rather by some miracle—man had dropped the idea of violent revolutions—not even to think of wars or Governmental upheavals of the dictatorial, suppressing type—provided all this were at present the case, and people went on as in the past, merely hoping and wishing and discussing, but still continuing to bear traditional but needless burdens—*one might well shudder at the hopelessness of any early or effective improvement of social conditions.*

I cannot refrain from pointing out again and again that all the precious institutions of democracy, including the possibilities of a certain individualism, and all the factors leading to ' inner freedom ' and to ' spontaneity ', and similar qualities of a higher human development—and added to all this the broadest public education appealing to the higher dispositions of man—all this together cannot and will not bear social fruits of a sufficient character if not firmly and continuously supplemented by forceful public measures, by *better planning of the social process.* The latter alone is capable of modifying human tendencies, which are based on inborn elementary instincts and on habit and traditional thinking.

2. No vote of the majority itself, no numerical oracle, whether originating in the ' genuine will ' of the voters or based rather on forceful propaganda—not even the ' free will ' of millions—can be a really justified and dependable factor in determining communal affairs. Solely the aspect of the possible maximal well-being of the possible maximal number of individuals and of families, through conscientious utilization of given means, ought to be the supreme measure of all necessary Governmental activity.

It is rather amazing how the world on the whole still continues on traditional lines ; though certainly reformatory ideas, as expressed here in a scientific psychological way, must be present in every average mind that meditates calmly and, as far as possible, independently on the vital aspects and questions of communal and individual life. But little substantial and systematic social progress has ever sprung from the spontaneity of the masses. Do not let us go on craving for, and merely restoring, previous institutions ; whilst disregarding the intrinsic formula of progress, and the absolute necessity of more daring conceptions, which present themselves implicitly in the course of history to the student of the social sciences.

It looks as if we were enemies of ourselves. We do not seem to realize the operation in larger communal spheres of the same *self-destructive instinct* which, as we know, is operative in the individual, and which destroys so much potential happiness of the individual—and of whole generations. We are not sincere guardians of ourselves. We know so much, and surmise even more ; we feel quite clearly that there should be a large, a very substantial revolution in men's minds, putting an end for generations to want, both physical and mental, to wars and bloody revolutions, to much useless exploitation. We feel that all this *could be—as it will be—reality one day*, in a perhaps very distant future. We feel that we need only make it an insurmountable, supreme law, that the *even distribution of burdens*—if not of means—without the traditional going in for politics, chauvinism, without that ' individual freedom ' which menaces the happiness of others—*ought to be the spiritual principle of governing.* There is nothing Utopian in this. The natural individualistic and aggressive tendencies of man could still find outlet enough. And on the other hand, many are the legal limitations and the conventional restrictions to which nowadays, as always in the past, even the most powerful squire, and the richest capitalist, and the most tyrannical ruler has had, at any rate, to submit and has had to allow to be an intrinsic part of his life.

Man is fitted with the sense of adaptation, and he is able to bear more or less restriction and accept guidance and social constraint. There is no necessity to break the core of the individual and to destroy all his spontaneity. But instead of insisting on the uncurtailed operation of the pressure of sheer traditionalism, of politics and over-acted nationalism, of social customs of no up-to-date significance, man should be relieved from a great part of these burdens, and placed instead under increased obligations and restrictions, serving a better and a juster communal life. The present author is convinced that in the end most people would readily accept this exchange of social burdens ; and only a few constitutionally ' asocial ' persons and socially difficult psychopaths would have to be denied their peculiar spontaneity, for the sake of the well-being of millions of fairly normal and adaptable human beings.

CHAPTER XXVI

SUGGESTIONS ON GENERAL REFORM

1. BEFORE embarking on the elaboration of a few suggestions as to a more ideal Governmental system and as to social reforms,

I wish first to restate the gloomy knowledge of all times as expressed already in Genesis : " The wickedness of man was great, and every imagination of the thoughts of his heart was only evil." [1] " For the imagination of man's heart is evil from his youth." [2] This, essentially, means that if left alone, man, the crown of creation, with all the gifts of his creative intelligence, and in spite of all his potential inclinations and genuine cravings for ethical and social improvement—man is insensible, ' infantile ', the prey of his irrational, instinctual, and emotional urges. His ' free will to be good ', his factual capability of becoming at least better, never works without external force, never operates sufficiently and successfully without external legislation and executive communal organization.

2. The spiritual foundation, the supreme principle of State-organization and management, must be of the highest possible standard of social humanity, according to the knowledge and insight attained by the particular generation. And the valid system of laws ought to contain the appeal, not less fundamental, to each subsequent generation and its Governments, to be constantly at work in creating social progress and improving the humane character of the governing State-principle. *Traditionalism and continuity of legality should be made for ever a crime, if there are clear indications of possible progress.* There cannot be, there must not be, any other essential foundation, permeating the particular legislation and executive power of the Government, than the supreme physical, emotional, and spiritual good of the greatest possible number of citizens.

And if the hard necessities of international events, for longer or shorter periods, may compel the Government to employ and organize the powers and resources of the State for overcoming acute danger—i.e. menace from without or within to the well-being of the nation—and if such necessities may require the suspension of the peace-time method of management of State-affairs, there will always be the possibility of mobilizing the population for this end. And undoubtedly such times will find a citizen better fitted for this end. But even if conditions of international tension should require strict conditions of emergency, for a whole generation, making well-nigh impossible the realization of increased human happiness, that should not prevent an ' ideal ' governing principle as suggested above from becoming

[1] Gen. vi. 5. [2] Gen. viii. 21.

supreme law and remaining in operation in the limited fields open to it.

3. The State is intrinsically responsible for the existing public opinion, for the extent of openly expressed prejudice and of manifest anti-social behaviour of innumerable people. It is the State's duty, because it is in its power, to exert active influence on public opinion in a socially more desirable direction. Education toward ethical thinking is as much a duty of the State as its practical development in the individual is the task of the individual. Incidental manifestations of State-ministers and judges, declaring that the official attitude favours justice, peaceable behaviour, and intellectual fight against prejudice, are simply futile gestures. A democracy that permits the free development of a prejudiced and aggressive spirit may end by becoming almost as bad as dictatorship.

If repression has to exist, if people have to exert a certain self-restraint, *let the main object of this repression be the aggressive, anti-social tendencies in man.* The experiment of a State-managed education toward the elementary, broad-minded principles of humanity, tolerance, and fairly unprejudiced thinking and acting is worth while. The State, with all the 'democratic' means at its disposal, could so spread a new public spirit that *it would become fashionable and reputable to think only on the lines of social decency.*

The Civil Servant, the teacher, the lawyer, the physician, the manager, all those called upon and 'licensed' to deal with the needs of their fellow-beings, should be strictly discouraged from manifesting any sort of prejudiced, or bureaucratic, or bullying and exploiting behaviour. Any sign of such a mentality should bring public disrepute, and disapproval from the State authorities; and should militate against advancement.

By such means the State would have created a very valuable stratum of population; and the social influence of this stratum would certainly spread the same humane mentality. No doubt, any education based mainly on the reward of public esteem, and on the threat of environmental moral pressure, is essentially a repression. We have, however, to wait and see whether the consequences of such repression reveal any harm to the mental balance of men, comparable to the obvious harm of the moral and economic pressure exerted on the majority of people under the existing system and its ideologies.

4. Freedom of the individual in his private life is one of the highest goods the State can allow. But the environmental conditions have first to be shaped in such a way as to enable the masses to enjoy the experience of inner freedom. This can only be effectuated by well-planned State pressure on over-individualistic and over-aggressive tendencies. Yet, as suggested in the course of this exposition, there is in man a healthy sense of submission, collaboration, tolerance—provided that there does exist a planned and just social process which induces the personality to develop on these lines. In the end, men will probably be fairly happy to have been moulded into peaceful and social human beings—much as the moody child, after having been forced to wash and to take his meal, becomes cheerful and happy, actually as the result of his 'improved' physical condition.

5. Work and productivity should be made not only the centre of actual living, but also the centre of 'emotional' social esteem. It is not meant to suggest by this any dictatorial labour-camps. But it is possible to create a mentality that frowns upon those who shirk working, and shows every sign of public approval and appreciation of those who do their best to spend their time usefully, and who try to recompense society for the order and protection they enjoy.

6. I think the State, in carrying out a substantial reform of social conditions, can help greatly to improve the institution of marriage. First of all, by giving more security to the individual, and more weight to everybody within the social organization, it will increase the personal prestige of man and wife not only generally but in each other's eyes too. Sexual attraction and emotional love are certainly strong buttresses supporting the factors of mutual esteem and mutual tolerance. But the more elementary layers of the psyche are greatly influenced by other factors too. If, for instance, the sexual factor, at a certain period of the marriage, recedes in intensity because for a time one partner does not look as attractive as usual, or because the other partner, for some subconscious reason, is at the time not fit to be attracted at all, then the non-sexual factors, such as personal poise or obvious self-confidence or cheerfulness and efficiency of the one partner, may help to shift the balance of sentiment in the mind of the other one into the positive, 'loving' direction.

The individual, if not deeply refined, is greatly influenced by the degree of ' strength ' shown by the other partner. Weak and ill and helpless people are pitied ; but the elementary layer of the mind does not respect them very much. And on the other side, strength and efficiency, and a certain impressiveness of the personality, may increase the sexual attraction. This is so chiefly in the sentiments of the woman toward the man. But it is just as possible for the man to be attracted by his wife if she enjoys a certain social esteem and he feels that *she is not unprotected* and not dependent on him both for her keep and for social esteem.

Mention should be made of a peculiar process that exists in our society, menacing the position of wives. The man professes to wish the woman pure, with plenty of inhibition in her sexual emotions, and with endless devotion to the well-being of her family. That is often the idea the girl or young woman gains before her marriage, from her intimate and wider circle. Then she marries, and automatically, perhaps without any conscious intention of hers, her psyche continues to develop the above trends ; it represses her genuine interest in her husband as lover, and sublimates all her interests into devotion to work and duty, whilst neglecting to cultivate her ' personality ' and ' sex-appeal '. In the meantime the husband grows in maturity, becomes older and more experienced—and at times, more or less even consciously, craves for a different, more ' vivacious ' wife. Usually he represses this wish, from self-esteem, and also from esteem for his wife. But the repressive process frequently fails, and nervous irritability appears, with the result that the man spends more time than is expedient for his family-happiness amongst other men ; at a club or in politics, at work, and so on.

The man enslaves the woman ; and then, when she unguardedly carries her self-denial too far, the man's emotions revolt against this. An improved social position of women may protect them from such a mistake.

7. Tolerance and adaptation is a function, a task, of the psycho-nervous system. Yet, if a person's mind is essentially disturbed—by worries, or simply by the sense of insecurity—or if a person has to spend his working time in an environment that shows no human regard for his personality, he may subsequently lack the mental energy necessary to carry out the task of adaptation and tolerance in his home. This, in turn, may, and frequently does, hurt the wife, decrease her wish to be attractive for him ; and

the process of deterioration of home conditions proceeds quickly, and reaches a stage from which there is hardly a way back. It is obvious where the significance of social reform comes in. And it is not only the *duty* of the State-organization to increase private happiness ; it is even in the *national interest* to have the energies of individuals and families protected from being used up in struggles with avoidable difficulties, and saved for the proper education of children, for communal work, and in general for gaining more and more cheerful citizens, men and women, for society. *It is a national advantage to have fewer embittered, cynical citizens, whose only interest is to compensate themselves for unhappiness by material advantages at the cost of others and of the community.*

Satisfactory family conditions require a certain amount of external 'supply'. One cannot, simply by will, and from a sense of duty, or for the sake of conventional interest, create love, tolerance, and the experience of happiness. Such tasks in our complicated time need the support of the community. And certainly there are many married couples who earnestly wish to cherish a peaceful, monogamous atmosphere within their mind and in their home—but they urgently need help ; and can only properly shape their lives relieved from the burdens of existence inherent in our social system.

8. Children need more protection than they enjoy today. Though it is not only the duty, but the natural right, of parents to look after their children, to decide upon their particular upbringing, their moral conceptions, religious tuition, pleasures, and so on—it is certain that many parents discharge this duty, and enjoy their possessive rights, in a way and to a degree that is harmful for the children. Boarding-schools, or schools where children could spend practically their whole day, should be available for all children who need a kinder or a stricter or a more quiet and more dignified environment, than their parents are able to give them. First of all, children need education in a healthy discipline ; but without threats, without destroying their personality, without employing the terrorism of superstitious or fanatical moral conceptions. The State has to exert its influence as much as is possible and permissible, to remove children from a family in which they are too much at the mercy of embittered and moody strictness on the part of their parents. Naturally, the State would not interfere with any specifically coloured religious education ; only where it appears obvious that the children are unduly unhappy,

and their mental development seems to be endangered. Much tact, much humanity, and much unbiased thinking may be needed for the individual decisions to be just and appropriate ; since, under our civilization, we cannot but admit the right of the parents to teach their children the ideology in which they themselves sincerely believe, as the only right one, as the only source of spiritual blessing.

The increased help which the State may give to families in education may contribute also to a part-solution of the phenomenon called fixation of the individual on to his parents. This complex follows *not only* automatic intra-mental difficulties of the child in breaking away and developing into an independent individuality ; a great part in the development of this complex is due to the attitude of the parents. They are gratified by the emotiona adherence and devotion of their children. *And the more they have had to toil for the child, the more they may feel that they are entitled to have the child for themselves.* And on the part of the child, the factor of *conscience* may prevent the desirable development of the psyche toward freedom, since the sense of gratitude and the awareness of owing almost everything to the parents may interfere with the healthy tendency toward independence.

We know that there is always repressed resentment against parents in the psyche of the child ; and the ensuing subconscious sense of guilt may join hands with the gratitude, and an undue attachment to the parents may then develop. It is easy to see that an improved and increased State-education may decrease such neurotic traits. The parents may, if self-critical, refrain from impressing themselves too much on their children. And the children may have *one ground less* for their neurotic fixation. We must not forget that every individual has a more or less accentuated awareness of his individual insufficiency, as a continuation of the weaker position of the child in the world of adults (Adler's ' inferiority feeling '). Educational conditions should at any rate tend to decrease and certainly not to increase it. In the long run the children are grateful to their parents and educators for allowing them to grow independent in mind and feelings—as a rule, more genuinely grateful than for a neurotically soft and emotional family atmosphere, in spite of all its warmth and snugness and shelter.

And children need more guidance and education in appreciating beauty and the various finer arts than they are given today. Infinite can be the refining influence of art on an individual who is so much attached to his own music or painting, or acting and reciting, as to feel unhappy without enjoying his particular kind of art regularly. Much aggressiveness, much superfluous interest in sex and politics, and in adventurous enterprises, could be eliminated from the life of youth by the ' sublimizing ' effect of art.

Youth has the right to be thoroughly educated about the serious spheres of sex, love and emotion in general, and in the elements of mental health, as established by the modern standards of science. Books in libraries, or occasional lectures for voluntary attendance, constitute an insufficient solution. To begin with, books on psychology and on the sex problem are, unfortunately, not often written by individuals free from ideological bias. Naturally, everybody should have the opportunity of knowing also about the controversial points on this matter. But there are certain objective facts which should be taught, more or less regularly, to young people ; these should be compelled to attend a few such lectures given by experienced, unbiased, highly qualified scientists, or by teachers specially fitted for such important tasks, on which much private happiness and much social interest may depend.

9. The ages which enslaved the child, and took the personality of the adolescent insufficiently seriously, have gone ; they have gone for ever. Increased refinement of individual life and improved conditions in general, rendering physical life easier, and above all the increased valuation of human freedom, have been followed by a better appreciation of the child and the adolescent. Social psychologists and educationists may have various logical explanations to offer for this fact. The present writer, however, believes that the phenomenon has one very substantial root : the adults are allowed, and given an opportunity, to enjoy their individual life, and the beauties and marvels of Nature, more than in the past. Consequently they are less inclined to grudge youth its freedom, and the mental ease resulting from its inexperience in the serious spheres of human life. In other words, there is less disguised hatred and aggression on the part of the parents and teachers. The past strictness and under-estimation of youth was largely a *hatred-neurosis*. And it is simply untrue that the child of our generation has become essentially less dutiful and less appreciative of his parents and of what they do for him. The attachment—the free attachment of spontaneity—experienced by the child of today toward parents and teachers is, on

the whole, perhaps even deeper; it is, at any rate, more frequent than in the last century. All counter-arguments referring to the risks of spoiling the child and to the alleged detrimental effects of leniency in education are simply mistakes or biased statements. The psycho-analysts know how real is the actual attachment of modern children to their parents, and how shaky is the foundation and how heterogeneous the psychic content of the manifested devoted attitudes of children of too strict parents. There is always much hatred in the background in such cases.

Childhood and youth are not merely preparatory phases for the life of the adult. They constitute on the average a third of life And this substantial part of human life deserves full appreciation. There is nothing less justifiable than the attitude that considers only the period of physical superiority and of economic independence in the life of the individual to be deserving of attention, and regards it as a privileged position. It is the duty of the State to bring home to the people this new educational principle. Unfortunately only a small fraction of mankind is given an adult life of fair pleasantness. Even if our economic conditions were twice as good as they are, the inevitable complications in the course of adult life, such as family troubles, illnesses, and the inevitable disappointments as to the attainment of early ideals and aims—all these things prevent general happiness of the adults. Yet the overwhelming majority of youth could be fairly happy. And here, there cannot be a social and educational reform too far-reaching, a benevolent consideration of youth too extensive. I repeat: the attitude of society toward children and youth is highly expressive of the greater or lesser amount of hatred operative in the subconscious spheres of the individuals. And there is nothing that better *repays* society than the tolerance and loving-kindness extended to the child and adolescent. A man can never be very bad, very asocial, if he bears within his mind a substantial amount of pleasant and happy recollections of his early years.

10. The advantage for a community comprising in itself the greatest number of healthy and able-bodied citizens has always been recognized. The militant State has needed physically fit soldiers. And the working community has required workers with sufficient strength and endurance. But the aesthetic aspect of the body has always been a sphere of life left to voluntary and private care. However, the advantage of a pleasant exterior in

every walk of life is so obvious that this point, too, merits the attention of those who are called upon to deal with public health. People tolerate better certain deficiencies of their fellowman and fellow-worker if he is for them a source of a little grace and attraction. They have internally to overcome a certain amount of displeasure, and irritability, if they are made to live and work with individuals who represent in their exterior and their gestures the concretization of disharmony. Such less fortunate people too easily evoke in the subconsciousness of others a process of 'complex-stimulation' [1]; i.e. their minor or major physical deficiencies become subconscious reminders to others of their own disapproved and condemned pathological 'complexes'; and consequently these others feel more uneasy about the unfortunate fellowmen than is justified by the little clumsiness or disharmony of features of the latter. It is the 'clumsy and disharmonic' sector of the onlooker's subconsciousness that experiences a repercussion and is the ultimate source of the irritable displeasure.[2]

Every child should thus have a claim to participate in all progress of 'cosmetic medicine and surgery'. First of all comes, naturally, the prevention of all disfiguring illnesses, however insignificant from the usual point of view of general health; then appropriate care for the teeth and complexion, and appropriate training of the muscles, of the gait and gestures in general. All this ought to belong to the elementary factors of school hygiene. And not only for a few 'chosen' children.

And it is not mere poetical sentimentalism when the author reminds the earnest reader of the happiness of parents at the sight of their nice-looking children. Existence appears to them more worth while, the extensive duties of private and social life more pleasurable and less burdensome, and, following this, their working capacity becomes better supported.[3] And, last but not least, the continual presence of their attractive children can make for a mutual toleration of those minor or major faults of each other in the life of many married couples.

It is perhaps even a pity that parents and children alike have to hurry and leave home in the early morning hours, when body and mind, and the whole personality, appear at their best, and that they are not afforded the opportunity of enjoying each other's existence. The author visualizes, indeed, a future stage of society when work and production will be more a matter of communal

[1] *Complex* is an active subconscious content.
[2] This has been proved by dream-analysis.
[3] Cf. Ch. VI, pp. 30, 31; and Ch. XII, pp. 69, 71, 73.

justice than of struggle and dependence ; and when it will not interfere so greatly and so cruelly with the genuine aim of life—the individual's family happiness and free self-expression.

11. The necessity of protecting the employee's economic condition has been duly recognized by all planners of a prosperous and democratic State-regime. What has, however, been neglected, because not clearly visualized, is the necessity of protecting the employee's personality. So long as the right of every individual to be free, and to feel free, is not seriously acknowledged, and this insight unequivocally displayed by appropriate legal measures, we still live in the ages of slavery. The employer, be it the State or a company or a private individual, must not be the oppressor of the soul of his fellowmen. But up to now he has been so, if he has not made a special point of not being so.

Approximately five per cent. of the persons with a nervous breakdown whom I used to see as consulting neurologist of a big ' panel ' in my home-country, the members of which were ' white-collar workers ' and employees of large business firms, traced their nervous breakdown to the constant strain caused by unpleasant superiors.[1] It is not a small thing to spend eight hours of the day, for years on end, in an unpleasant environment, having to submit to the authority of a superior whom one cannot appreciate, or who happens to be of a neurotic or a paranoid type. Under the existing conditions it is not advantageous to an individual to change the place of his occupation ; his possible loss in advancement, and even of pension in some countries, is too serious to be risked by any individual, and especially by a father of a family.

Think of a man of the better-educated type, with a well-developed personality, who is compelled to flatter a dull superior for years, for decades—simply for the sake of bread : a heart-breaking situation, a shame for our enlightened period. The opportunity must be given to such an individual to change his job, without any harm to his existence, in order to meet his craving for a more cultured and human environment. And any complaint against a manager—whether private or public—should be carefully examined, and appropriate steps should be taken to save the private happiness of his subordinates. A man has the right to come home, after his day's work, with full self-confidence, with unbroken mental independence, with joy of life and with

[1] The number of cases where this factor contributes to neurosis is greater, but many people repress its realization.

energy enough to live for himself and for his family. Such a social reform is within easy reach. To forestall the operating of subconscious pathological complexes is only an ideal aim, never possible to attain in full for all people. But to give to *every individual* who has to bear the inevitable social burden of being a subordinate as much relief from environmental pressure as is *in fact possible* should be a serious concern of any truly human democracy.

12. The desirable increase of the social sense in people, and the appropriate particular attitudes of the individual, need not be created ' from nothing '. This reformed social condition would not represent a new, additional burden on man's mind and nerves. There exists already much ethical sense and a widespread ethical attitude, cultivated by the individual occupational strata. To mention only a few instances, in order to illustrate what is meant by the above suggestion—the associations of lawyers, medical men, clergymen, educationists, and also of business men and craftsmen in relation to their customers, all these and other occupational groups have developed and cultivated a special ' professional ' ethic, which in its analysis is distinguishable from the intellectual interest of the occupation, to do one's job properly. There is therefore ethical spirit and will, and, if one may use the expression, ' ethical energy ' in plenty.

All that would be needed is a modification, a ' switching over ' of these attitudes and energies to fit in better with the modernized social conceptions ; and so to enable the individual to feel genuinely at ease within the modernized social frame. There is an important point to stress. The usual socialistic arguments have mostly viewed the problem of the employee. This was justified in the past by the concrete conditions and necessities. Today the problem has grown considerably both in extent and in complexity. The members of the individual occupational strata still possess more or less the past ideology of their group ; and they devote all their efforts, though unsuccessfully, to maintaining it, protecting it in the face of rapidly changing economic and social conditions. The social position of the physician, for instance, can no longer be the same as it was fifty years ago. That air of unapproachable authority, enjoyed by the doctor of the past, no longer appeals as a rule either to patients or to physicians. Above all, this superiority no longer possesses dynamic enough to maintain itself, owing to the gradually growing necessity for the doctor to fight for his existence, and to take part in that exciting race of competition which is initiated by the progress of science, and by the larger degree of specialization. This latter fact makes people more critical, and causes them to increase their claims on the members of the profession. New difficulties and tasks, though with a quite different background, seem to face other occupational strata too. It is obvious to anybody that the general type of clergyman has had to undergo a substantial change in the direction of closer intimacy with his parishioners. And to find the members of this highly conservative profession amongst those who are calling for a reformed, socialized world, testifies also to my thesis. All this means new specialized fields of study for the social psychologist. This task is comparable to the modern science of industrial psychology, devoted to the vast problems connected with modern industrial life, a special field of psychology which has made so good a start in Great Britain.

13. The attentive reader will have understood that the present writer has not in mind an absolutely communistic State. First of all, we have to await the further development of the U.S.S.R., whilst carefully watching and learning, and applying in our countries what we have seen and learned, as much as is expedient. But even if one were inclined to advocate Communism, one could not justifiably waste even one page in a small volume for this end ; since it is obvious that the individual countries of Europe and America are at present not prepared to accept a true copy of Russian conditions.

However, the author regards an intensified State-control as unequivocally necessary : a control of all spheres absolutely essential to a high level of well-being of the citizen. But, first of all, he advocates the absolute protection of the individual ; of all individuals, and not only of those who are clever or competitive enough. The State-organization should enable the millions of citizens to develop and to live as individuals free from unnecessary pressure, whether from external or from internal, i.e. neurotic, sources. I do not regard such a state of affairs as Utopian ; at least, not so far as concerns the material possibilities utilized in the State-organization.

It need not be said that the author's idea is not a dictatorial penal code of increased severity, but a gradual change in official and public opinion about social and anti-social behaviour. The discouragement of all the wrong in this direction should be mainly left to the moulding *social process*. And the start of this change can be made only by the Administration. It is not possible for everybody, however high his position, to be totally just and benevolent and free from human weaknesses and prejudices. But as the judge in Great Britain puts on his wig and gown when performing his sacred duties, so any member of the Administration could put on such a ' mental wig and gown ' when dealing with the lives of others. To leave, however, to the voluntary fairness of the individual such wide spheres of decision beyond the possibility of control does not seem to be truly democratic, if this implies the care for the happiness of all benevolent members of a State-community. To rely on the spontaneous fairness of a few implies inevitably a considerable risk of harmful individualism on the part of those others who are of a different mental make-up. The best path to a gradual remedy appears to be, as pointed out repeatedly in this book, a planned improvement of public opinion and of the general *social process* that creates the social character of the individual, whether a simple citizen or a member of the Administration.

14. The legal system of a State requires an appropriate budget and an appropriate staff for carrying it out. It may be asked how a theoretician, elaborating his plans of social improvement at his writing desk, can suggest a hypothetical ideal of State-management, which—if taken seriously—would involve at least the creation of a new, very large department for the physical and mental well-being of the nation.

Well, the theoretician has his ideas also about this. He is firmly convinced, and this has been stated by others in the past, that the existing administrative body could be substantially simplified ; and that a not inconsiderable amount of rules and regulations, of formal requirements in jurisprudence and local administration, could be dispensed with. The lawyer will probably disagree. The average lawyer is so fond of the accumulation of details he once learned, and which he daily employs, that he would hardly be prepared to give up even a fraction of them. Yet, let him consider how many details of minor significance are temporarily—for instance, for the duration of the war—dispensed with. He knows much more than the psychologist of the historical genesis of individual regulations ; how many legal formalities are only sacred because they are sanctified by the passage of time ; how many exist only because there is a continuous need to alter and to supplement the 'primary' legal definitions and regulations, which are not themselves absolutely up to date and are not absolutely necessary for beautifying our present mode of life.

No doubt the new, reformed State-idea, the new and supreme department for social well-being, would necessitate a great administrative system, both scientific and executive. Yet, as has been said above, much of what appears to the conservative lawyer and politician as absolutely necessary in the existing administration could be dispensed with.

15. It is impossible for any individual country—and especially for the many small States in Europe—to prevent wars, and pressures of a less bloody character exerted on them from outside. But it is absolutely possible for them to enjoy internal prosperity more than in the past, if they are granted years of external peace. It is definitely possible to create a more humane, more quiet, more productive and more progressive atmosphere within the State. And it is not improbable that such enviable internal conditions may at the same time command some respect in the hearts of people living in other countries and under less progressive conditions. The immediate or distant effect of such appreciation may perhaps bear political fruits not obtainable for a small country by the best armaments and fortifications.

It would be short-sighted, and even criminal, to rely again on democracy alone, as this principle has been conceived in the past. Political democracy, as we know, is incapable in itself of guaranteeing internal peace and the happiness of all its citizens, *if* the spiritual background of the mass of the people is *not* based on the absolute acknowledgment of humanity, social justice, and condemnation of prejudices. And this is never the case spontaneously! To accomplish this task, a stronger hand will have to be employed, and a management of internal affairs different from the usual conceptions. We know today, more or less well, what is the necessary amount of 'freedom' of the individual to make him genuinely happy and to make him enjoy the life within the community. It is not the freedom that gives a free hand to hate-propaganda, to the many 'anti-ideologies', or encourages a continuous fight for political aspirations that spring simply from different tastes and group-interests.

16. I have to recall here a remark made at the beginning of this

work, about the reluctant attitude of the 'efficients' toward minute analytical social research or toward 'socialistic' suggestions. Those people who are in 'a good position', and a great number of those who read much and have enough initiative to view with a critical mind what they read, and to argue in writing and in public speeches against suggestions of reform, belong in fact to the small fraction of the population that is fit to live fairly successfully under existing conditions. Their fitness, whether based on personal toughness or, incidentally, on the better circumstances of their private lives, has been the very factor that has helped them through all the existing handicaps, and permitted them to become and to be what they are, in spite of all the social deficiencies weighing on others. They may simply argue that we reformers exaggerate, that we are too sensitive, or even paranoid [1] personalities; and that the existing order, with some additional small allowances to the masses, may be just the right state of affairs.

Others, psychologically more gifted, may realize that we have in mind the weaker but larger strata of society; and may think that it is, in fact, not worth while, for their sake, to reform society; just as we wish the neurotic to become 'stronger', and to adapt himself to the standards of the 'normal', and not vice versa. The reader, if not acquainted with the broader and detailed facts of social life, may even think that the present writer, being a physician to the psychopaths and neurotically weak, is drawing from his material of research general conclusions that by no means justify the generality of his argument.

My reply is the following: True, we need and advocate the various fields of social reform for the benefit of those millions who are at present not happy enough, not efficient enough, but who are still very human, and potentially very estimable specimens of the genus *homo sapiens*; and who, if put into a different social and ideological setting, could constitute more distinguished, and even more productive, members of the human community; apart from the fact that they are morally, at any rate, entitled to have more human happiness and ease than they actually happen to enjoy, if this be possible.

The absolute number of those who participate in a more or less quiet, more or less dignified and peaceful but still stimulating life of the human communities, could be substantially greater if our social conditions, economic and cultural, were more advanced. And I declare that the great majority of those who today are

[1] Cf. Ch. XV, p. 91.

unable to view with sympathy and understanding the possible change of their accustomed modes of existence, will gladly accept it if once in operation. I am reminded of an aged gentleman, once a very successful business man, but a tyrant over his environment, and now a poor refugee in Great Britain, but still no less insistent on imposing his will and opinion on his people. His son, himself well over forty, and hard-working, wanted to buy a wireless-set. True, their means were very limited ; but the air of depression weighing heavily on the younger members of the refugee family—poverty, restriction of movements, relatives tortured abroad—fully justified the desire for a little entertainment. But the 'tyrant' said definitely : "I will not have it." Then, a year later, somehow the old man had to agree ; I do not know exactly why. First only grudgingly watching the 'younger generation' listening to the English broadcasts—he himself hardly speaks a few words, being now about eighty-five —little by little he took possession wholly of the wireless ; and now there is no part of the day when he is not listening to anything available. And he is proud of the wireless-set "he had bought". Something similar may happen with our 'conservatives at any price', both young and old, both rich and only moderately well-to-do, if they be allowed to live in a world basking a little more in the warm and bright sunshine of an obviously reformed communal condition.

17. There would still remain millions of backward people, sluggish, indolent and simple, and unable to enjoy and participate in higher standards ; though nobody need suffer from hunger, from lack of a proper roof, or from oppression. But there cannot be that mathematical equality advocated by unrealistic pedants, or by lazy and inefficient but rather aggressive demagogues, who themselves and whose followers were incapable of contributing in the slightest degree toward communal interests and communal harmony. That marked inequality of human living obtaining today is not wrong because of the very fact of inequality, but only because society needs a little more means and rights for millions, and cannot achieve this without taking something from the privileged few ; but not simply in order to create an artificial equality, and to satisfy the envy which lies disguised behind such tendency for a 'social symmetry'. There will always be, and has to be, some means of enabling those who are capable of utilizing the extra for a better cultural and human standard,

whether that of their fellowmen or of their own family, to have access to some 'extra allowances' of life; necessary, for instance, for research, for art, or necessary for meeting their more sensitive needs of body and mind, and so on. But simply to equalize means and to give a superfluity for free use to people who would not know what exactly to do with their rights and means, apart from spending more, such a state of affairs is certainly not the guiding idea of the present author. Consequently, he claims still to be a realist, though of that second kind mentioned in his introduction.

I am satisfied that people, deep down in their mind, do not want 'equality'; this notion is a more or less artificial concept, created in response to social difficulties. So far as individual psycho-analyses lasting for several months can indicate, the only thing people want is subjective happiness; it is their neurotic trend that makes them more or less want to *submit others*, preferably their nearest relatives, to their 'prestige'. At the same time, even this latter trend does not exclude the absolute readiness on their part to *submit to others*. There is no genuine trace of an elementary urge for 'equality'.[1]

But the even distribution of means is not the fundamental principle leading toward true social improvement. One should rather say that the *more even distribution of burdens and pains*, both private and communal, is the desirable magic formula. And this latter is quite a different matter. It implies rather less pressure on the poor and uninfluential, the abolition of the continuous fear about elementary needs of the individual and his family, that is, the abolition of that sense of insecurity by which—it is true—you can rule and keep down the free individuality of millions. What is also necessary is the maximum of knowledge on vital problems of psychology and sexual character; the granting of all available means of public assistance, to forestall the development of an advanced neurotic make-up or physical disability; and also an appropriate share for everybody in the beauties of civilization and nature. And the enjoyment of all this should be made possible without much bureaucratism, without making the individual into a dependent child, into a docile subject of Governmental charity.

The complexity and the difficulty of materialization of such a standard is clear to everybody, the present writer included. And the only possible thing to do, for our generation, is to start immediately with acknowledgment of the necessity of such an aim, and to bring about at least the manifest spirit of such a

[1] The urge for 'equality' and prestige springs largely from neurotic sources.

State-idea in the needlessly complicated organizatory mechanism existing today all over the world.

On the whole, what I advocate aims essentially at the maintenance of more or less protected privacy of every life. I have in view the possibility of private enterprise, besides the necessary State-control of all goods essential for human life ; and also a firm State-control safeguarding the individuality, the inner freedom of a person who is employed, whether by the State or by a private firm.

The world *can* be managed without such human ideals ; everything can be maintained as it is, if only a strong police force prevents wars and the violence of revolutions. *People are weak, if not given the opportunity to be strong.* They have their faculty of adaptation. They could still tolerate existing conditions. They could laugh and live, as they have done so far. And they might learn again to forget the idea of a social reform, forget to visualize the possibility of altering so much which is not absolutely necessary to put up with. They could be deceived again, kept in ignorance and in unawareness of what could be done for them and for all of us. *The question is only whether it is just, whether it is human, and whether it pays to prevent, for decades, the earlier materialization of that which is at a later period bound, inevitably bound, to come.*

CHAPTER XXVII

CLOSING REMARKS

1. At the end of his expositions the author feels that he has to add a few explanatory words as to the objective validity, or, let us say more modestly, as to the fair probability of his statements, interpretations, conclusions, and suggestions. He thinks that the psychological part of his present work is based on fundamental findings, on which there cannot but be a more or less general agreement amongst the eclectics.[1] The particular method of his presentation, and a number of new interpretations of his own, do not, he thinks, essentially alter this fact.

As to the social aspect of his expositions, there is a need for saying the following : The author has not in mind a particular

[1] Scientists choosing the best from different sources, and not dogmatically committed to one school of psychology or philosophy.

country and Government, least of all Great Britain alone. He happens to know a few countries in Europe ; and he has now, for four years, been staying in Great Britain. He has had the opportunity of analysing a sufficient number of people from different countries, and of different occupational strata of the working and the middle classes, to feel his conclusions on the whole justified. He is satisfied that the aspects discussed by him, in their totality, apply more or less to conditions in Europe, but this latter taken as a whole ; though certainly not to the same degree, in all points, to each part of Europe. He has to admit, for instance, that the sense of ' fairness and courtesy ' and that calm leisurely way of living, both peculiar to the social life of Great Britain, make things, for the most part, easier in actual life. And this fact may induce a great number of people to believe that the social suppositions on which this work is based do not apply at all to this country. He also admits that the religious life of this country has contributed on the whole rather beneficially than not to general conditions. He would, however, find it unfair to deny the little information his book may give, especially to the reader of this country. It is not the separate individual points, but the whole frame of this book, that he would like to receive consideration and to stimulate discussion. There is much in his work, though deficient, which may merit, and find, the genuine interest of the public. Psycho-analyses, carried out on people in this country, show that in the way of expressing life there may be a substantial difference between people of this country and those in other European countries. But the fundamental psychic processes, problems, conflicts, and their environmental sources, appear essentially identical all over Europe. And with this, the possible methods of remedy may, perhaps, also be substantially the same. *The main thing is to grasp the essence of phenomena.* And the main idea of this book is : *Do not let us rely, in the great cause of human happiness, on the voluntary fairness of people alone, if there be a way of intensifying, through a better-planned social process, this fairness of spirit in all inter-human relations.*

The highly complicate conditions of a just distribution of opportunities of living require much mutual consideration, limitation of the individual's movements, and the creation of a well-organized community. But the author is convinced that the ultimate aim of all social progress should be the integrity and satisfactory condition of the affect-self of the individual. Man's emotions, their harmony and their full expression, as far as possible, on refined lines of living deserve the protection of the social organization. And the latter is, in fact, not worthy of existence except as a means of enabling the individual human being to ' be ' and to enjoy his unique being. All endeavours to deny the significance of the individual and his right to live, and to put first a communal organization for its own sake, are, so the author feels, expressive of disguised hatred : hatred of self and of others based on an unjustified, neurotic inferiority-complex of individuals. The given conditions at any period of history might require maximal restrictions of the individual's life ; but the awareness of their forced necessity should never cause to disappear from consciousness the genuine aim of life : the individual's freedom to self-expression and self-experience. To allow again such a mistake on this point, and even to organize it, would again pave the way for slavery, would lead to the mental self-destruction of the millions, and to the tyrannical power of a few. In the sphere of bodily well-being there has never been a mistake about what is ' normal ' and desirable. Pain and suffering, and limitation of the duration of life, are, in fact, constant untoward accompaniments of human existence. But the clear awareness about what is the ideal of desirable normality has never been doubtful to the sane mind.

2. The attentive reader must have realized that the core of the social problem is the element of aggression in its various aspects and manifestations.

Resentment, envy and hatred, competition and exploitation, educational and ' conventional ' pressure, intimidation by prejudice, superstition, and ill-conceived moral conscience, the gross inequality in social significance—these are the individual chapters of the treatise on aggression. The impulse of hatred in the individual interferes in various fields, and under various disguises, with the life of the others ; and through unsuccessful repression the emotion of hatred recoils on the personality, and produces disease, malfunctions of body and mind. This is perhaps the most significant truth discovered by psycho-analysts. And the counter-force and remedy of this destructive tendency has also been unequivocally established. It is *love*.[1] Not that love which only gives, not that love which gives itself up. It is rather the love that enjoys its loving. The enjoyment of oneself through fair satisfaction with oneself, and, to even a greater degree, the enjoyment of others who are the object of human love, are the

[1] Cf. Freud, *Civilization and Discontent* ; Stekel, *Sadism and Masochism.*

factors which keep in balance the excess of aggressive and ' self-aggressive ' tendencies. The faculty of love does not depend merely on will. It depends first of all on the presence of lovable objects ; and then on the absence of mental complexes inhibitory to its operation. One cannot love oneself if, rightly or not, dissatisfied with oneself. And one cannot love others if to do so entails too much risks of being disappointed, under-estimated, and burdened with obligations which break one's individuality—and finally one's faculty of love. Our existing social system exposes the feeling of love in friendship, marriage, and family to constant attacks. It makes the individual neurotic, irritable, insincere, intimidated ; in brief, unfit for a life of adaptation. The warm atmosphere of the family circle is at the same time permeated with tension and suppressed hatred. All social collaboration and personal friendship is overshadowed by the cloud of distrust. Religion and the moral code not only lift the mind into the heights, but press the personality down on its knees. And in this life-atmosphere the love-satisfaction decreases, and the hatred impulse, though suppressed, increases. What manifests itself as unbridled sexuality is in fact a symptom of mental unrest, of unquenched thirst for love, for satisfying love.

The diagnosis is made. The pathogenic factors are discovered. The aim of treatment appears clear. But the particular ways and means are still in obscurity. Man should be relieved from every avoidable pressure, and enabled to love. But how to attain this aim ? Where to start with constructive demolition, where with new building ? How to forestall the volcanic manifestations of transition ? There is no full, no clear answer possible today. But the aim is clear ; and this itself is reassuring.

Reformatory attempts, whether political, social, or religious, have always met with considerable resistance. The bias of tradition, habit, and tangible interests, in brief the powerful influence of existing conditions (*social process*) on men's minds, result as a rule in the firm belief that suggested changes are neither desirable nor feasible. This subjective attitude of inertia is objectively and intensely opposed by the accumulation of historical experience. Innumerable conceptions at first considered to be Utopian dreams, or even expressions of inacceptable and dangerous tendencies, have ultimately become part and parcel of universal ideologies ; again and again advocates of new doctrines, once attacked as enemies of social morality, have become admired leaders ; so that it is rather naïve at any time of history to view existing conditions with any confident belief in their final validity. The richer our historical and scientific experience has grown, and the more frequent has been the occurrence in the course of social and scientific history of sudden and revolutionary changes, the greater should be the doubt felt by any generation and any individual in the objectivity or finality of the existing system of beliefs and conceptions. The overwhelming lesson of historical experience should create a new attitude in thinking men toward their contemporary mode of seeing things. If anything is clearly taught by history, it is the relativity of particular human conceptions and modes of social life. There are obviously only two fixed principles : the undesirability of avoidable human burdens and suffering ; and the logical duty of each generation to explore every avenue that promises improved material and spiritual life, both social and individual. The writer thinks that nothing can be more fundamental than the acknowledgment of this truth, apparently so simple ; and there should be hardly anything in the social and cultural life of men that is weighty enough to have superiority over the before-mentioned two fundamental principles.

3. Now here arises a serious practical problem. Just as the individual is entitled to adhere to conditions and principles that make him fairly happy, so each generation is fully entitled to value and cherish those traditions and ethical principles which contribute to the welfare and happiness of the substantial majority of its members. No doubt this fact might stand in the way of progress for the future. But it must not be allowed to do so. There must be a mode of wise compromise between a firm adherence to contemporary social and moral philosophy on the one hand, and the regard for a possibly different future on the other. The same conflict—and a similar compromise—has taken place from time immemorial in the life of parents with regard to the later independence of their children. There must be a mode for the present generation to live its life fully, combined with an allowance for the different needs of the future, social and cultural. One may live peacefully in one's own home, and live there after one's own fashion, without interfering with the freedom of the pathways leading into the distance. This is, of course, only a very simple analogy. And no analogy, even the best, fits exactly. But the principle of a wise compromise is nevertheless fully valid. It is the most obvious teaching of man's cultural and social history.

A substantial part, however, of the masses in all countries cannot imagine a mode of life essentially differing from that of past centuries. For innumerable people—both people with personal initiative and those of an inert and dependent type—social and national life means restless competition, struggle, and the exploitation of those in weaker positions in all fields. In view of these undeniable facts, it may appear very doubtful whether increased knowledge and the craving of merely passive or even of ethically minded masses will ever create a new world. We know a number of people who like studying in solitude, or discussing with friends, modern social conceptions and deep philosophical problems, individuals who at certain moments—on holidays as a rule—unmistakably display even metaphysical inclinations ; but when they return into the prosaic life of everyday activity, to business, politics, communal affairs, they return with the greatest naturalness to the usual *savage modes* of thinking and valuing, essentially the modes customary since time immemorial amongst the mass of ' non-idealists '. They even do not realize the contradiction in their attitude ; they do not realize that their ' lofty moments ' are not only an implicit condemnation of their normal life, but pointers to a feasible different way of feeling and acting.

Here is, indeed, one of the puzzles of human nature, which may make the critical mind doubt whether increased knowledge may be conducive to progressive social improvement. And indeed, the writer himself has no other logical suggestion to offer than to say : The greatest possible knowledge and the greatest possible improvement of social organization, in brief the greatest gift of kindness manifested on the part of a State to its members, cannot have the desired effect without ruthless suppression of anti-social, inert, destructive tendencies on the part of those who essentially are savages in modern clothes, speaking the language of ' the ascent of man ', and employing the advances of human science, for the gratification of their traditional ' subcultural ' modes of living.

Let us keep in mind that human beauty and health are ' natural ' notions ; but their concrete existence has to be cultivated and safeguarded throughout life. Still more has social progress to be continually protected. Traditional modes of life are dynamic, not only because firmly based on the foundation of habit ; but especially because they are more apt to give easy gratification to savage, aggressive, and self-destructive tendencies. Let us not deceive ourselves about this psycho-biological factor in man's history. It is not the intellect, neither is it the idea of a spiritual soul, that is the main moving factor of life ; these are but forceful correctives, and directives pointing to a distant idealistic goal. *Consequently, there cannot be a smooth and voluntary maintenance of human achievement.* There must be a firm and militant defensive attitude, if there is to be a substantial degree of life to be lived. And similarly, let us not forget another socio-psychological fact. Aggression, and achievements attained through power and force, exert a peculiar attraction on men's minds ; not only in the Far East, but, in fact, in deeper layers of the psyche of Western dwellers too. And these ' deep ' layers are even not necessarily very deep. Finally, let us repeat what has been explained in one of the previous chapters : Any individual or any organization of individuals in executive power who are indifferent or tolerant toward the slightest sign of social aggression are in fact granting satisfaction to their own half-conscious criminal tendencies. It is too late when their indulgence has led to developments they did not wish.

A substantial part of the usual State-administration in the past was nothing but such organized destruction of human individuality and happiness. Hundreds of thousands of people were considered ' Stateless ' and either simply tolerated or limited in their elementary rights, or even shifted from frontier to frontier. And all this occurred without serious necessity for the well-being of those who did possess the scrap of paper testifying to their uationality or ' naturalization '. I have to state that the conservative Great Britain has been far ahead of all other modern countries in human toleration of foreign people who were no proven enemies of the State or of society. And the prosperity of the others, and the general standard of life, seem not to have suffered but rather to have gained in consequence of this tolerance of what has been in fact an enrichment of the autochthonous population by different elements.

I cannot help stating the following : Social organizations breed all that is good and all that is evil. The implicit spirit of the State in its legal aspect and administrative practice becomes ultimately the fertile soil of destructive movements, emerging within that piece of Earth. This statement, though daring, is based on an acknowledged thesis of psycho-pathology. I have pointed out more than once in the course of this book : Neurotic phenomena are essentially only distortions or disproportionate magnifications of subconscious tendencies, present also in the normal. And similarly, pathological traits of character are in fact distorted imitations of existing and approved social attitudes. *But it is not the 'distortion' alone that makes the normal abnormal, and transforms the approved into the not approved.* The normal and approved contains in itself the nucleus of the abnormal and not approved. The social organization itself prepares, as it were, for times that are favourable for manifest terror and destruction, the conditions for development of these manifestations. A State-organization which would persistently try to weed out corruption, exploitation, passive or active participation in aggression, could therefore never become a fertile soil for destructive manifestations, however great the influence from abroad might be.

4. And now, after having finished his work, the author would like to say a few words about some apparent deficiencies of it. The reader, if enthusiastic about a new and better life in the immediate future, may miss concrete proposals regarding methods of 'sublimating'[1]—or eliminating—those aggressive tendencies of man so much in the fore of discussion today, and so horrifyingly manifested now for some years. The present writer does not feel qualified to expound on such practical proposals. There are others, more experienced in the study of concrete social spheres, who are called upon to give their lead to their contemporaries. Besides, it will be agreed that once the mental background has started to remodel itself, the feeling and thinking of people will spontaneously create such fields of activity as, apart from their usefulness, will help to 'abreact' (neutralize) those hating and aggressive feelings. Only the spheres of actual living can suggest and bring into being such definite modes of activity. The chief task of the scientific and political leaders is to do their best to give a socially beneficial impetus and direction to the minds of people.

Other remarks of many a reader may refer to apparent contradictions, revealed to the attentive critic of this book. He may not, for instance, grasp fully the compatibility of a broad interference by the State, as advocated by the author, with that democracy and freedom so much discussed, and with that spontaneity and that individual colouring of life which has been so much approved of in this book. Yet this very instance of contradiction may illustrate the general answer of the author. In describing mental attitudes, it is quite possible to stress the importance of two different factors, both equally valuable, both equally desirable for the refinement and 'socialization' of man.

[1] Cf. Ch. VIII (6), (7), (8), pp. 38-40 ; Ch. X, p. 52 ; Ch. XI (6), p. 66.

To employ a very simple analogy, acid and alkaline [1] compounds are equally needed by the living cells. Human behaviour, whether in individual or communal life, is always the result of many simultaneous, and at times contradictory, mental tendencies. (The neurologist is reminded of the 'final common pathway' of Sherrington ; this notion expresses the fact that the anterior spinal roots, directing the muscular actions, are the collectors of different impulses coming from various brain centres, which multifarious impulses, as it were, vie for the possession of this final common pathway.) And this is the author's essential reason for presenting his exposition in small chapters, each reviewing a separate field of human life ; instead of writing a book of a more coherent composition. For practical purposes, the understanding of such circumscribed domains of individual and social life is definitely more expedient than the usual academic continuity of exposition, which leaves no gaps in the presentation of its subject. And this selective and separating mode of description may present the appearance of certain inconsistencies between the individual statements of the present author ; but these apparent contradictions, so he dares to say, are essentially non-existent.

He also favours the more or less essay-like journalistic fashion for his *Social Psychology*. And he rather regrets that some of the chapters [2] *had* to be written in the difficult phraseology of psycho-analytical and academic psychology. If his capacity for clear and easy presentation in English had been more accomplished than is, in fact, the case, he would, with great pleasure, have discussed even these more difficult topics in the easier, popular way. Because a true social science, destined for practically minded people, does well to abandon the abstract and lengthy modes of scientific presentation, in favour of a description approaching the actual, realistic ways of thinking and seeing, usual in ordinary life.

[1] In terms of chemistry, *antagonists*.

[2] They present some new suggestions to the student and research-worker of psychology. The author asks his colleagues too to pay some attention to his small volume.

APPENDIX

EXPLANATION OF A FEW PSYCHOLOGICAL CONCEPTS

Bisexuality of the human individual is a psychological notion. In the sexual sphere it implies that every person has the potential faculty to feel in a libidinal way towards members of the same sex. Besides, many men display feminine attitudes ; whilst a number of women would like to be in certain respects men. The libidinal bisexuality is a cerebral function ; it is not directly the result of the heterosexual hormone that is present in the organism of each individual. Folliculin, the ovarian hormone, can always be found in the testes and urine of adult males. Androgene, the male genital hormone is also excreted in the female urine, and thus its presence in the female organism is certain.

Dreams are products of unconscious activity during sleep. Their contents are mainly disguised, symbolic representations of mental problems of that person. The various organic processes have their share in the stimulation of dreams ; but they do so through creating or intensifying emotional processes. In the opinion of the author, dreaming is an emotional process contributory to mental health. It goes on throughout sleep, but it does not result always in recollectable dream-pictures.

Instincts are innate biological drives, prompting the individual to feel, desire and behave in a definite manner without previous educational training. The instincts of self-preservation, of procreation, of pugnacious self-defence, the instinctive curiosity to explore anything new in one's environment, the parental love and care for the offspring, etc., are such innate biological drives. It is clear that their particular operation is greatly subject to individual variations, such as are due to moulding influences of society and education, in brief, to human cultivation. And this makes human instincts essentially different from the parallel forces in animals.

Another characteristic of these drives in man is that their operation is *not* limited to the attainment of necessary biological goals. The instinct of sex, aggression, curiosity, and the desire for food, are certainly operative far beyond the corresponding biological necessity. It is intellectual and intentional suppression, followed by subsequent intra-psychic repression, that sets a limit to these urges in their manifestations as ' appetites ' and wish tendencies.

Intravert (self-centred) is the type of individual whose emotional interest and thinking is in a great degree concerned with his own subject, physical and mental. He has a difficulty in feeling with and for others (*empathy*=putting oneself into the other's position) ; he can only insufficiently participate in general interests, to react in the ways of average people, and to conceive of himself as one of the multitude.

Such an individual is subject, more than is expedient, to the influence of his subconscious, unrealistic tendencies. And external reality does not sufficiently counteract and modify his own individual sentiments. (The expression '*autistic*' denotes a similar concept.)

Another difficulty in escaping from the undue influence of one's subconscious processes is the result of a certain narrowness of outlook. The broader one's outlook or intellectual latitude, and the more adaptable one's emotional thinking, then the more limiting and modifying are those factors which interfere with the influence of subconscious processes. This applies particularly to the process of *projection* and formation of prejudiced—logically unassailable—opinions. Such a narrow outlook is frequently the outcome of a defective development of the emotional function as a whole ; and it is in many such individuals associated with other signs of unsuccessful repression of instincts. A certain type of moral education stressing too much the 'devil in man' appears greatly to increase the factors leading to such a development.

Extravert denotes the alert, social and practical type of personality. If an extravert type shows the signs of intellectual and emotional limitations just described, he probably suffers from the presence of too strong pathological complexes with no sufficient counter-regulation.

Neurosis and psychosis are two different conditions, and *not*—as the layman believes—the second a stronger form of the first. In the neurosis there is a disturbance in subconscious ideation, owing to an emotional disturbance (conflict). But we do not assume that the chemical functioning of the brain is substantially altered in neurosis. The neurotic always knows that his abnormal feelings or obsessional ideas are the expression of an illness. Besides, a very great number of neurotic subconscious disturbances create merely 'organic complaints' (felt in the heart, alimentary tract, head, etc.).

The psychotic (in popular language the 'mental patient') suffers, so it is thought, from a substantial disturbance of the chemical processes in the brain. The various delusions, and loss of critical intellect, are the consequence of this basically 'physical' abnormity. The psychotic always believes in the reality of his delusions. He is unable to do differently ; we say : he has no insight into his condition—apart from very light cases. The treatment of psychosis is thus primarily physical, not psychological. *The true neurosis is not the forerunner of psychosis.*

It is, however, true that the analysis of delusions of true psychotics contributed much valuable information to psycho-analysis. On the other hand, the understanding of dream symbols enabled the psychiatrist to understand many of the delusions of psychotics. But it has to be pointed out once more—the delusions are not the essential illness of such a patient. A similar case is the alcoholic who speaks and behaves improperly ; all this is only due to the poisoned condition of his brain. The delusions are subconscious contents, brought to the fore following the psychotic disturbance of brain-processes. These psychotic conditions are at present treated by electric convulsions, by insulin-coma, or prolonged sleep induced by drugs.

Normal and abnormal with respect to mental functioning are not two opposite kinds of processes. With Freud and Bleuler we believe that, essentially, all that is manifested in neurosis or psychosis is only the distorted or over-accentuated contents and tendencies present in the healthy, in the ' normal.' Bleuler states : " Hence what is important, we shall only recognize from the study of the growing psyche of the child, and above all from aberrations of those already developed in psycho-pathology. *At this time one of the most important, if not the most important path to a knowledge of the human psyche is by way of psycho-pathology* " (*Psychiatry*, Ch. XII).

' Normal ' and ' healthy ' are adjectives applicable to a person who is capable of an average subjective satisfaction, enjoying the average gifts and pleasures of life, having an interest in an appropriate measure of work, and being able to live a life of mutuality with a number of other people. It is the ultimate balance of all intra-mental processes, the fair proportioning of part-tendencies, that decides a person's ' normality ' and subjective well-being. But the quality of tendencies is universally equal in all human beings. Thus, a person may behave in his dreams in a manner he would never consciously choose to do. And there are always so-called ' abnormal ' complexes in the normal too, but only in a dormant, subconscious and counter-regulated state.

Reaction means response. In psychology—and in general physiology—it denotes thus not a simple passive reflex. Reactive formations of the mind are complex products, in response to a certain life-situation. If, for instance, one has had a disappointing experience with a friend, he may develop the idea that 'most friends are unreliable', and that one ought to be very cautious in trusting anyone. Clearly, this is a newly formed mental attitude of a complex nature; or more accurately, it is a complex mental content, together with a tendency to behave in a certain manner. It is obvious that in the course of life every individual acquires a great number of similar reactive formations, both of a useful and of an unjustified character. What we call *experienced behaviour* is in fact that which is based on an accumulation of such useful reactive formations. A great number of reactions are only of a temporary nature; they do not repeat themselves in the same way in the course of life. Every individual has, however, a number of characteristic constant reaction patterns.

Subconscious processes of the mind are indispensable for health. It is only their incidental disturbance that leads to neurotic manifestations. And such disturbances are in the life of many people as unavoidable as are indispositions of their physical organs.

LIST OF BOOKS

List of a few books which the author happens to know, that deal with individual items discussed also in the present work. Since the expositions of the present author are in no way based on the works of these other authors, the reader may certainly gain added view-points and information from their perusal.

J. C. Flugel, *The Psycho-analytic Study of the Family* (Hogarth Press), 1921.

This work contains a comprehensive analysis of the family and of related spheres of life. It is based on a very effective utilization of a vast literature. Hundreds of references to the problem, scattered in psycho-analytical publications, chiefly of the Freudian circle, are elaborated into a homogeneous whole, and enriched by the author's comments.

The psychological background of the work consists in the main in the classical conceptions of psycho-analysis (libido-theory, Oedipus-complex, etc.) ; and it is probable that in a new edition today the author would increase the value of his remarkable work by presenting additional new aspects of individual and social psychology. However, it is certainly still modern enough to merit the attention of all engaged in social and educational research.

J. C. Flugel, *Sublimation*, in the Br. J. Ed. Psychology, 1942.

This paper is the most up-to-date presentation of the problem known to me. Its references to related publications are well-nigh exhaustive, and its reasoning is convincing through its scientific objectivity.

Erich Fromm, *The Fear of Freedom* (Kegan Paul), 1942.

This work tries to account for the readiness to accept dictatorship, and even oppression, by the feeling of ' isolation of the individual ' in our age, which may be followed by a genuine ' fear of freedom '. The author speaks also about the *social process*, the problem of sadism and masochism, and about the position and responsibility of the individual in a true democracy of freedom.

Ad. Lowe, *The Price of Liberty : A German on Contemporary Britain*, 1937.

The author in his pamphlet says clever things on individualism, collectivism, and on that spontaneous collectivism which alone is compatible with freedom of the individual.

Karl Mannheim, *Diagnosis of Our Time* (Kegan Paul), 1943.

This book comprises a number of well-written essays on a variety of social and cultural problems. Attention may be drawn especially to the chapters on ' Mass Education and Group Analysis ' and ' Christianity and the Planned Democratic order '.

PETER NATHAN, *The Psychology of Fascism* (Faber and Faber), 1943.

This small volume contains a graphic description of the phenomenon of prejudice and its psychological foundation, *i.e.* the projection of self-contempt and self-hatred on to others.

KAREN HORNEY, *The Neurotic Personality of Our Time* (Kegan Paul), 1937.

This author, for a great number of years member of the traditional Freudian school and an experienced psycho-analyst, attempts to modify Freudian conceptions in the light of Adlerian theories. The neurotic manifestations and analytical complexes are brought into relation with general social phenomena, assigning a role of priority to the latter.

INDEX

For Product Safety Concerns and Information please contact our EU representative GPSR@taylorandfrancis.com
Taylor & Francis Verlag GmbH, Kaufingerstraße 24, 80331 München, Germany

www.ingramcontent.com/pod-product-compliance
Ingram Content Group UK Ltd.
Pitfield, Milton Keynes, MK11 3LW, UK
UKHW021955180926
475701UK00003B/50

9781138875777